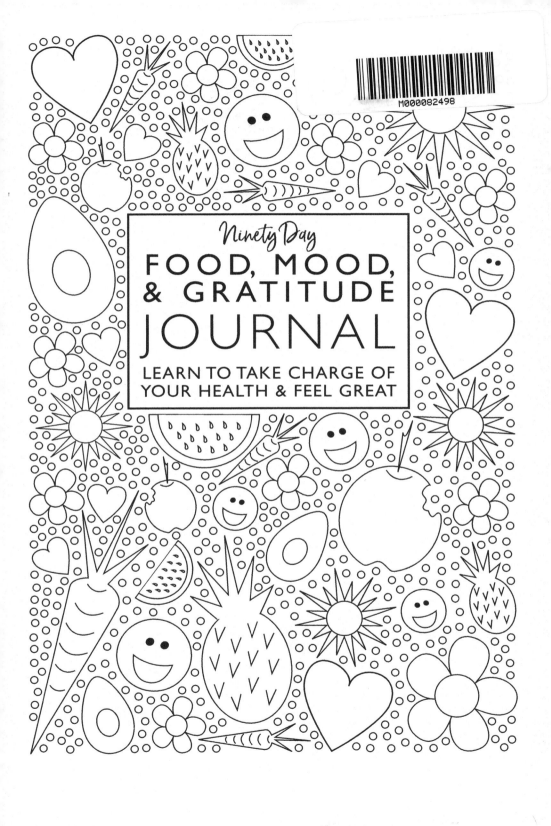

Ninety Day
FOOD, MOOD, & GRATITUDE
JOURNAL

LEARN TO TAKE CHARGE OF
YOUR HEALTH & FEEL GREAT

Published by Ingenium Journals
Toronto, Ontario, Canada M6P 1Z2
All rights reserved.
ingeniumbooks.com

Cover design and interior art: Heidi Hackler

ISBN: 978-1-989059-41-8

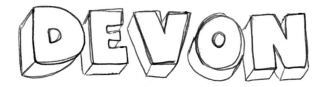

Dedicated to my nieces and nephew,
Annika, Noelle, Sarah-Jane, and Tate.
May your lives be full of happiness and wellness.

WHY USE A *FOOD, MOOD, & GRATITUDE JOURNAL?*

Keeping a *Food, Mood, & Gratitude Journal* is a great way to kick-start your health and wellbeing. With this journal, you can be a wellness detective, tracking clues and piecing them together for your optimal health.

Sleep is a key component to overall mood and health. Tracking how well you slept each night will start to give you clues to improve your sleep and health habits.

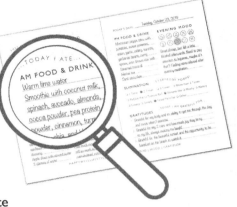

Did you know that **food and mood** are directly related? Your gut is always communicating with your body. Your gut microbiome plays an integral role in this system, and the molecules of what you eat communicate with your brain, pretty cool, huh?!

Most of your serotonin (your happiness neurotransmitter) is produced in your gut too. What you eat can directly affect your serotonin production. If you eat something that you are sensitive or allergic to, your body will let you know in subtle (or not so subtle) ways. Tracking food and mood can give you further clues to create optimal wellness.

Your **elimination** system is one of the main ways your body detoxes. Everybody poops! Though most people don't want to talk about their poop, looking at your stool provides clues to your overall health and wellbeing. Pay attention.

Finally, daily **gratitudes**. Research shows writing down three things each day you're grateful for improves your overall happiness, which ties in directly to health and well being.

This *Food, Mood, & Gratitude Journal* will help you track your overall health and wellness and better understand where to consider making diet or lifestyle modifications.

TAKING A DEEPER LOOK AT THE
FOOD, MOOD, & GRATITUDE JOURNAL

HOW DID YOU SLEEP LAST NIGHT?

Sleep is one of the biggest factors affecting overall health and wellness. And most people don't get enough sleep, or don't sleep soundly when they do sleep. So tracking your sleep habits can be very beneficial to overall wellness.

LAST NIGHT I SLEPT... _____7_____ HOURS

● Like a Rock   ○ Restless   ○ Difficulty Falling Asleep

○ Woke up tired   ○ Woke in the night   ○ Woke 2-3 times

Good quality sleep is a vital part of overall wellness. In fact, sleep has been shown to:
• Improve memory
• Contribute to a longer life span
• Reduce inflammation
• Improve athletic performance
• Improve grades
• Sharpen attention and help avoid accidents
• Aid in weight loss

Here are some ways you can improve your sleep:
• Turn off all blue light (ie: screens, phones, TVs, tablets) one hour before bed
• No caffeine after noon
• Rub lavender essential oil on the bottoms of your feet before bed
• Eat a kiwi or drink tart cherry juice before bed
• No food or alcohol for three hours before bed
• Avoid exercise in the late evening
• Try a guided meditation or a Yoga Nidra meditation

WHAT DID YOU EAT TODAY & HOW DO YOU FEEL?

By keeping track of what foods you eat each day along with how you feel mentally and physically, you can start to see patterns and correlate which foods may be adversely affecting you mentally and physically.

Do you notice any of the following symptoms?
- Frequent sleepiness or brain-fog after eating a certain food, like wheat?
- Congestion after eating dairy?
- Do certain foods seem to cause canker sores?
- Do you experience gas or bloating after a meal?
- Any unresolved skin rashes?

None of these are "normal" reactions to eating. And symptoms like these can indicate a food intolerance.

If you start to feel certain moods or physical symptoms that you'd rather not be feeling, listen to your body. It knows best. You may be eating something your body isn't so keen on.

Try cutting those foods out for a couple of weeks and see if it helps. Sometimes eliminating just one or two foods from your diet can make a world of difference to your overall health and well being.

If you eat to support your gut microbiome (not your taste buds that have hijacked your brain!) your body and brain will be much healthier.

...TODAY I ATE...

AM FOOD & DRINK
Warm lime water
Smoothie with coconut milk, spinach, avocado, almonds, cocoa powder, pea protein powder, cinnamon, turmeric, ginger, chia, and blueberries.
Herbal tea

...TODAY I FEEL...

MORNING MOOD

I was tired and cranky when I got up this morning, but after meditating and playing with my cats I felt better! But I felt a bit bloated after the smoothie??

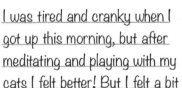

WHY IS PROPER ELIMINATION SO IMPORTANT?

The body has three main ways to eliminate toxins: through the stool, urine, and sweat. And while you might never have given much thought to your stool, it can give you big clues to your overall health and wellbeing. So it's a good idea to pay attention to it.

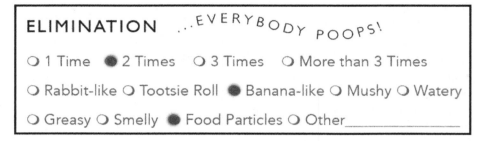

Did you know it's normal to poop two or even three times a day? Once a day is a minimum for most people. If stool matter sits around in the intestines the body starts to re-absorb those toxins. And that's never a good thing.

If you find yourself constipated (going less than once a day, or having hard-to-pass stools like rabbit-poops or tootsie rolls) try some of these ideas:
• Drink more water. (Caffeine and alcohol are both dehydrating, so if you drink those, you need to up your normal water consumption.)
• Take a mineral supplement at bed time that includes potassium and magnesium to help optimize movement of the intestines.
• Exercise more regularly, especially aerobic exercise or movements that get your gut moving.
• Eat more fiber in the form of veggies and fruits with skins on.
• Pay attention to the food/mood section. Unresolved food sensitivities can cause constipation.
• Meditate to unwind and de-stress. Stress is directly linked to constipation.

If you poop more than three times a day, that can be a sign of an overactive colon, irritable bowel syndrome, or food sensitivities. Whole food particles in your stool can indicate poor digestion or leaky-gut. And greasy stools can indicate that your liver, gallbladder, or pancreas aren't doing their job.

WHAT ARE YOU GRATEFUL FOR?

Writing down three gratitudes each day can significantly improve your overall happiness, health, and well being. Thinking them or saying them is great too, but the most powerful happiness-boost comes from writing them down.

Think outside the box when you write your gratitudes. It's easy to be grateful for your spouse, kids, pets, or life. But how about being grateful for your ears that hear so well, or your knees that let you run, or for the opportunity to help the little old lady with her groceries?

GRATITUDES ...TODAY I AM GRATEFUL FOR...

1. Grateful for my body and its ability to get me through the day, and move when I exercise.
2. Grateful for my 2 cats and how much joy they bring to my life, always making me laugh!
3. Grateful for the beautiful sunset and the opportunity to be barefoot on the beach to watch it.

Congratulations on buying this Journal! You've taken the first step towards reaching your optimal wellness and happiness goals.

Now that you understand the WHY behind tracking your *Food, Mood, & Gratitude* (plus sleep and elimination!) you'll be better able to piece together the clues to your happiness and wellness, and make healthier choices.

To Your Health!

P.S. If you like to color, I created the cover and title page just for you, enjoy!

MONTH ONE

FUN FACT:

80%

...number of Americans who do not get the
recommended seven-eight hours of sleep a night.
Sleep deprivation is linked to weight gain.

LAST NIGHT I SLEPT...   <u>   8.5   </u>   HOURS

cold / flu symptoms
O Like a Rock   ● Restless   O Difficulty Falling Asleep

O Woke up tired   O Woke in the night   O Woke 2-3 times

...TODAY I ATE...   ...TODAY I FEEL...

AM FOOD & DRINK   ## MORNING MOOD

- Coffee silk
  creamer   😃 🙂 😖 🙁 😣
- apple & almond   😮 😐 😕 😣 💤
  butter

                                          sick @ work

MID-DAY FOOD & DRINK   ## AFTERNOON MOOD

- veggies & hummus   😃 🙂 😖 🙁 😣
- turkey stick   😮 😐 😕 😣 💤
- veggie straws
- cookies   sick @ work

- Jamba Juice
- 2 packs saltines

TODAY'S DATE: _____january 9th 2020_____

PM FOOD & DRINK

_____
_____
_____
_____
_____
_____
_____

EVENING MOOD

😃 🙂 😐 🙁 😫

😯 😌 😕 😣 💤

_____
____sick and very____
____tired____
_____
_____

ELIMINATION ...EVERYBODY POOPS...

○ 1 Time ○ 2 Times ○ 3 Times ○ More than 3 Times

○ Rabbit-like ○ Tootsie Roll ○ Banana-like ○ Mushy ○ Watery

○ Greasy ○ Smelly ○ Food Particles ○ Other_____

GRATITUDES ...TODAY I AM GRATEFUL FOR...

1._____
_____
_____

2._____
_____
_____

3._____
_____
_____

FOOD | MOOD | GRATITUDE   13

LAST NIGHT I SLEPT... _____ HOURS

O Like a Rock   O Restless   O Difficulty Falling Asleep

O Woke up tired   O Woke in the night   O Woke 2-3 times

...TODAY I ATE...

AM FOOD & DRINK

_____
_____
_____
_____
_____
_____
_____
_____

MID-DAY FOOD & DRINK

_____
_____
_____
_____
_____
_____
_____
_____

...TODAY I FEEL...

MORNING MOOD

_____
_____
_____
_____

AFTERNOON MOOD

_____
_____
_____
_____

TODAY'S DATE: _____

PM FOOD & DRINK

_____
_____
_____
_____
_____
_____
_____

EVENING MOOD

😀 🙂 😐 🙁 😧
😮 😕 😖 😣 😴

_____
_____
_____
_____
_____

ELIMINATION ...EVERYBODY POOPS...

○ 1 Time   ○ 2 Times   ○ 3 Times   ○ More than 3 Times

○ Rabbit-like ○ Tootsie Roll ○ Banana-like ○ Mushy ○ Watery

○ Greasy ○ Smelly ○ Food Particles ○ Other_____

GRATITUDES ...TODAY I AM GRATEFUL FOR...

1._____
_____
_____
2._____
_____
_____
3._____
_____
_____

LAST NIGHT I SLEPT... _____ HOURS

○ Like a Rock   ○ Restless   ○ Difficulty Falling Asleep

○ Woke up tired   ○ Woke in the night   ○ Woke 2-3 times

...TODAY I ATE...   ...TODAY I FEEL...

AM FOOD & DRINK

_____
_____
_____
_____
_____
_____
_____
_____
_____

MORNING MOOD

(faces)
(faces)

_____
_____
_____
_____
_____

MID-DAY FOOD & DRINK

_____
_____
_____
_____
_____
_____
_____
_____

AFTERNOON MOOD

(faces)
(faces)

_____
_____
_____
_____
_____

TODAY'S DATE: _____

PM FOOD & DRINK

_____
_____
_____
_____
_____
_____
_____
_____

EVENING MOOD

😃 🙂 😐 🙁 😰

😮 😕 😬 😖 😴

_____
_____
_____
_____
_____
_____

ELIMINATION ...EVERYBODY POOPS...

○ 1 Time   ○ 2 Times   ○ 3 Times   ○ More than 3 Times

○ Rabbit-like ○ Tootsie Roll ○ Banana-like ○ Mushy ○ Watery

○ Greasy ○ Smelly ○ Food Particles ○ Other_____

GRATITUDES ...TODAY I AM GRATEFUL FOR...

1._____
_____
_____
2._____
_____
_____
3._____
_____
_____

LAST NIGHT I SLEPT... _____ HOURS

O Like a Rock   O Restless   O Difficulty Falling Asleep

O Woke up tired   O Woke in the night   O Woke 2-3 times

...TODAY I ATE...

AM FOOD & DRINK

_____
_____
_____
_____
_____
_____
_____
_____

MID-DAY FOOD & DRINK

_____
_____
_____
_____
_____
_____
_____
_____

...TODAY I FEEL...

MORNING MOOD

_____
_____
_____
_____
_____

AFTERNOON MOOD

_____
_____
_____
_____
_____

HAPPYWELLLIFESTYLE.COM

PM FOOD & DRINK

_____
_____
_____
_____
_____
_____
_____
_____

EVENING MOOD

😃 🙂 😐 🙁 😫
😮 😕 😕 😣 💤

_____
_____
_____
_____
_____

ELIMINATION ...EVERYBODY POOPS...

○ 1 Time ○ 2 Times ○ 3 Times ○ More than 3 Times

○ Rabbit-like ○ Tootsie Roll ○ Banana-like ○ Mushy ○ Watery

○ Greasy ○ Smelly ○ Food Particles ○ Other_____

GRATITUDES ...TODAY I AM GRATEFUL FOR...

1. _____
_____
_____
2. _____
_____
_____
3. _____
_____
_____

LAST NIGHT I SLEPT... _____ HOURS

O Like a Rock   O Restless   O Difficulty Falling Asleep

O Woke up tired   O Woke in the night   O Woke 2-3 times

...TODAY I ATE...   ...TODAY I FEEL...

AM FOOD & DRINK

_____
_____
_____

MORNING MOOD

_____
_____
_____
_____
_____

MID-DAY FOOD & DRINK

_____
_____
_____

AFTERNOON MOOD

_____
_____
_____
_____

TODAY'S DATE: _____

PM FOOD & DRINK

_____
_____
_____
_____
_____
_____
_____
_____

EVENING MOOD

_____
_____
_____
_____
_____
_____
_____

ELIMINATION   ...EVERYBODY POOPS...

O 1 Time   O 2 Times   O 3 Times   O More than 3 Times

O Rabbit-like O Tootsie Roll O Banana-like O Mushy O Watery

O Greasy O Smelly O Food Particles O Other_____

GRATITUDES   ...TODAY I AM GRATEFUL FOR...

1. _____
_____
_____

2. _____
_____
_____

3. _____
_____
_____

LAST NIGHT I SLEPT... _____ HOURS

○ Like a Rock   ○ Restless   ○ Difficulty Falling Asleep

○ Woke up tired   ○ Woke in the night   ○ Woke 2-3 times

...TODAY I ATE...

AM FOOD & DRINK

_____
_____
_____
_____
_____
_____
_____
_____

MID-DAY FOOD & DRINK

_____
_____
_____
_____
_____
_____
_____

...TODAY I FEEL...

MORNING MOOD

_____
_____
_____
_____
_____

AFTERNOON MOOD

_____
_____
_____
_____
_____

HAPPYWELLLIFESTYLE.COM

PM FOOD & DRINK

_____
_____
_____
_____
_____
_____
_____

EVENING MOOD

😃 🙂 😐 🙁 😫
😳 😖 😕 😣 😴

_____
_____
_____
_____
_____

ELIMINATION ...EVERYBODY POOPS...

○ 1 Time   ○ 2 Times   ○ 3 Times   ○ More than 3 Times

○ Rabbit-like ○ Tootsie Roll ○ Banana-like ○ Mushy ○ Watery

○ Greasy ○ Smelly ○ Food Particles ○ Other_____

GRATITUDES ...TODAY I AM GRATEFUL FOR...

1._____
_____
_____
2._____
_____
_____
3._____
_____
_____

LAST NIGHT I SLEPT... _____ HOURS

○ Like a Rock   ○ Restless   ○ Difficulty Falling Asleep

○ Woke up tired   ○ Woke in the night   ○ Woke 2-3 times

...TODAY I ATE...

AM FOOD & DRINK

_____
_____
_____
_____
_____
_____
_____
_____
_____

MID-DAY FOOD & DRINK

_____
_____
_____
_____
_____
_____
_____
_____

...TODAY I FEEL...

MORNING MOOD

_____
_____
_____
_____
_____

AFTERNOON MOOD

_____
_____
_____
_____
_____

HAPPYWELLLIFESTYLE.COM

TODAY'S DATE: _____

PM FOOD & DRINK

_____
_____
_____
_____
_____
_____
_____

EVENING MOOD

😀 🙂 😐 🙁 😧

😮 😕 😐 😣 😴

_____
_____
_____
_____
_____

ELIMINATION   ...EVERYBODY POOPS...

○ 1 Time   ○ 2 Times   ○ 3 Times   ○ More than 3 Times

○ Rabbit-like ○ Tootsie Roll ○ Banana-like ○ Mushy ○ Watery

○ Greasy ○ Smelly ○ Food Particles ○ Other_____

GRATITUDES   ...TODAY I AM GRATEFUL FOR...

1. _____
_____
_____

2. _____
_____
_____

3. _____
_____
_____

FOOD | MOOD | GRATITUDE

LAST NIGHT I SLEPT...

_____ HOURS

○ Like a Rock   ○ Restless   ○ Difficulty Falling Asleep

○ Woke up tired   ○ Woke in the night   ○ Woke 2-3 times

...TODAY I ATE...

AM FOOD & DRINK

_____
_____
_____
_____
_____
_____
_____

MID-DAY FOOD & DRINK

_____
_____
_____
_____
_____
_____
_____

...TODAY I FEEL...

MORNING MOOD

_____
_____
_____
_____

AFTERNOON MOOD

_____
_____
_____
_____

PM FOOD & DRINK

_____
_____
_____
_____
_____
_____
_____
_____
_____

EVENING MOOD

😀 🙂 😐 🙁 😢
😮 😌 😕 😣 😴

_____
_____
_____
_____
_____
_____

ELIMINATION   ...EVERYBODY POOPS...

○ 1 Time   ○ 2 Times   ○ 3 Times   ○ More than 3 Times

○ Rabbit-like ○ Tootsie Roll ○ Banana-like ○ Mushy ○ Watery

○ Greasy ○ Smelly ○ Food Particles ○ Other_____

GRATITUDES   ...TODAY I AM GRATEFUL FOR...

1._____
_____
_____
2._____
_____
_____
3._____
_____
_____

LAST NIGHT I SLEPT... _____ HOURS

○ Like a Rock   ○ Restless   ○ Difficulty Falling Asleep

○ Woke up tired   ○ Woke in the night   ○ Woke 2-3 times

...TODAY I ATE...

AM FOOD & DRINK

_____

_____

_____

_____

_____

_____

_____

_____

MID-DAY FOOD & DRINK

_____

_____

_____

_____

_____

_____

_____

_____

...TODAY I FEEL...

MORNING MOOD

😀 🙂 😐 🙁 😢
😮 😕 😑 😣 💤

_____

_____

_____

_____

_____

AFTERNOON MOOD

😀 🙂 😐 🙁 😢
😮 😕 😑 😣 💤

_____

_____

_____

_____

_____

PM FOOD & DRINK

_____
_____
_____
_____
_____
_____
_____
_____

EVENING MOOD

😃 🙂 😐 🙁 😫
😮 😖 😕 😣 😴

_____
_____
_____
_____
_____

ELIMINATION   ...EVERYBODY POOPS...

○ 1 Time   ○ 2 Times   ○ 3 Times   ○ More than 3 Times

○ Rabbit-like ○ Tootsie Roll ○ Banana-like ○ Mushy ○ Watery

○ Greasy ○ Smelly ○ Food Particles ○ Other_____

GRATITUDES   ...TODAY I AM GRATEFUL FOR...

1._____
_____
_____

2._____
_____
_____

3._____
_____
_____

LAST NIGHT I SLEPT...   _____ HOURS

○ Like a Rock   ○ Restless   ○ Difficulty Falling Asleep

○ Woke up tired   ○ Woke in the night   ○ Woke 2-3 times

...TODAY I ATE...

AM FOOD & DRINK

_____

_____

_____

_____

_____

_____

_____

_____

MID-DAY FOOD & DRINK

_____

_____

_____

_____

_____

_____

_____

...TODAY I FEEL...

MORNING MOOD

_____

_____

_____

_____

_____

_____

AFTERNOON MOOD

_____

_____

_____

_____

_____

_____

HAPPYWELLLIFESTYLE.COM

PM FOOD & DRINK

_____
_____
_____

_____
_____
_____
_____

EVENING MOOD

☺ ☺ ☺ ☹ ☹
☺ ☺ ☺ ☺ zz

_____
_____
_____
_____
_____

ELIMINATION ...EVERYBODY POOPS...

○ 1 Time   ○ 2 Times   ○ 3 Times   ○ More than 3 Times

○ Rabbit-like ○ Tootsie Roll ○ Banana-like ○ Mushy ○ Watery

○ Greasy ○ Smelly ○ Food Particles ○ Other_____

GRATITUDES ...TODAY I AM GRATEFUL FOR...

1._____
_____
_____

2._____
_____
_____

3._____
_____
_____

LAST NIGHT I SLEPT... _____ HOURS

○ Like a Rock   ○ Restless   ○ Difficulty Falling Asleep

○ Woke up tired   ○ Woke in the night   ○ Woke 2-3 times

...TODAY I ATE...

AM FOOD & DRINK

_____
_____
_____
_____
_____
_____
_____
_____

MID-DAY FOOD & DRINK

_____
_____
_____
_____
_____
_____
_____
_____

...TODAY I FEEL...

MORNING MOOD

_____
_____
_____
_____
_____

AFTERNOON MOOD

_____
_____
_____
_____
_____

TODAY'S DATE: _____

PM FOOD & DRINK

_____
_____
_____
_____
_____
_____
_____
_____

EVENING MOOD

😃 🙂 😐 🙁 😫

😮 😕 😐 😣 😴

_____
_____
_____
_____
_____
_____

ELIMINATION   ...EVERYBODY POOPS...

O 1 Time   O 2 Times   O 3 Times   O More than 3 Times

O Rabbit-like O Tootsie Roll O Banana-like O Mushy O Watery

O Greasy O Smelly O Food Particles O Other_____

GRATITUDES   ...TODAY I AM GRATEFUL FOR...

1._____
_____
_____

2._____
_____
_____

3._____
_____
_____

LAST NIGHT I SLEPT... _____ HOURS

○ Like a Rock   ○ Restless   ○ Difficulty Falling Asleep
○ Woke up tired   ○ Woke in the night   ○ Woke 2-3 times

...TODAY I ATE...

AM FOOD & DRINK

_____
_____
_____
_____
_____
_____
_____
_____
_____

MID-DAY FOOD & DRINK

_____
_____
_____
_____
_____
_____
_____

...TODAY I FEEL...

MORNING MOOD

_____
_____
_____
_____
_____
_____

AFTERNOON MOOD

_____
_____
_____
_____
_____
_____

HAPPYWELLLIFESTYLE.COM

PM FOOD & DRINK

_____
_____
_____
_____
_____
_____
_____
_____
_____

EVENING MOOD

😄 🙂 😐 🙁 😩

😳 😖 😕 😣 😴

_____
_____
_____
_____
_____

ELIMINATION ...EVERYBODY POOPS...

O 1 Time   O 2 Times   O 3 Times   O More than 3 Times

O Rabbit-like O Tootsie Roll O Banana-like O Mushy O Watery

O Greasy O Smelly O Food Particles O Other_____

GRATITUDES ...TODAY I AM GRATEFUL FOR...

1._____
_____
_____

2._____
_____
_____

3._____
_____
_____

LAST NIGHT I SLEPT... _____ HOURS

○ Like a Rock   ○ Restless   ○ Difficulty Falling Asleep
○ Woke up tired   ○ Woke in the night   ○ Woke 2-3 times

...TODAY I ATE...

AM FOOD & DRINK

_____
_____
_____
_____
_____
_____
_____
_____

MID-DAY FOOD & DRINK

_____
_____
_____
_____
_____
_____
_____
_____

...TODAY I FEEL...

MORNING MOOD

_____
_____
_____
_____
_____

AFTERNOON MOOD

_____
_____
_____
_____
_____

HAPPYWELLLIFESTYLE.COM

TODAY'S DATE: _____

PM FOOD & DRINK

_____
_____
_____
_____
_____
_____
_____
_____

EVENING MOOD

😀 🙂 😐 🙁 😫

😮 😕 😶 😣 😴

_____
_____
_____
_____
_____

ELIMINATION ...EVERYBODY POOPS...

O 1 Time   O 2 Times   O 3 Times   O More than 3 Times

O Rabbit-like O Tootsie Roll   O Banana-like O Mushy O Watery

O Greasy O Smelly   O Food Particles O Other_____

GRATITUDES ...TODAY I AM GRATEFUL FOR...

1. _____
_____
_____

2. _____
_____
_____

3. _____
_____
_____

FOOD | MOOD | GRATITUDE

LAST NIGHT I SLEPT... _____ HOURS

○ Like a Rock ○ Restless ○ Difficulty Falling Asleep

○ Woke up tired ○ Woke in the night ○ Woke 2-3 times

...TODAY I ATE... ...TODAY I FEEL...

AM FOOD & DRINK

_____

_____

_____

_____

_____

_____

_____

_____

MORNING MOOD

_____

_____

_____

_____

_____

MID-DAY FOOD & DRINK

_____

_____

_____

_____

_____

_____

_____

_____

AFTERNOON MOOD

_____

_____

_____

_____

_____

TODAY'S DATE: _____

PM FOOD & DRINK

_____
_____
_____
_____
_____
_____
_____
_____

EVENING MOOD

😃 🙂 😐 🙁 😫

😮 😕 😑 😣 😴

_____
_____
_____
_____
_____
_____

ELIMINATION ...EVERYBODY POOPS...

○ 1 Time   ○ 2 Times   ○ 3 Times   ○ More than 3 Times

○ Rabbit-like ○ Tootsie Roll ○ Banana-like ○ Mushy ○ Watery

○ Greasy ○ Smelly ○ Food Particles ○ Other_____

GRATITUDES ...TODAY I AM GRATEFUL FOR...

1._____
_____
_____

2._____
_____
_____

3._____
_____
_____

LAST NIGHT I SLEPT... _____ HOURS

○ Like a Rock   ○ Restless   ○ Difficulty Falling Asleep

○ Woke up tired   ○ Woke in the night   ○ Woke 2-3 times

...TODAY I ATE...

AM FOOD & DRINK

_____
_____
_____
_____
_____
_____
_____
_____

MID-DAY FOOD & DRINK

_____
_____
_____
_____
_____
_____

...TODAY I FEEL...

MORNING MOOD

_____
_____
_____
_____
_____

AFTERNOON MOOD

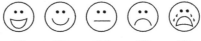

_____
_____
_____
_____
_____

TODAY'S DATE: _____

PM FOOD & DRINK

_____
_____
_____
_____
_____
_____
_____
_____

EVENING MOOD

😃 🙂 😐 🙁 😦

😮 😑 😕 😣 😴

_____
_____
_____
_____
_____

ELIMINATION   ...EVERYBODY POOPS...

○ 1 Time   ○ 2 Times   ○ 3 Times   ○ More than 3 Times

○ Rabbit-like ○ Tootsie Roll ○ Banana-like ○ Mushy ○ Watery

○ Greasy ○ Smelly ○ Food Particles ○ Other_____

GRATITUDES   ...TODAY I AM GRATEFUL FOR...

1._____
_____
_____
2._____
_____
_____
3._____
_____
_____

FOOD | MOOD | GRATITUDE

LAST NIGHT I SLEPT...

_____ HOURS

○ Like a Rock   ○ Restless   ○ Difficulty Falling Asleep

○ Woke up tired   ○ Woke in the night   ○ Woke 2-3 times

...TODAY I ATE...

AM FOOD & DRINK

_____
_____
_____
_____
_____
_____
_____
_____

MID-DAY FOOD & DRINK

_____
_____
_____
_____
_____
_____
_____

...TODAY I FEEL...

MORNING MOOD

_____
_____
_____
_____
_____

AFTERNOON MOOD

_____
_____
_____
_____
_____

HAPPYWELLLIFESTYLE.COM

TODAY'S DATE: _____

PM FOOD & DRINK

_____
_____
_____
_____
_____
_____
_____
_____

EVENING MOOD

_____
_____
_____
_____
_____

ELIMINATION ...EVERYBODY POOPS...

O 1 Time   O 2 Times   O 3 Times   O More than 3 Times

O Rabbit-like O Tootsie Roll O Banana-like O Mushy O Watery

O Greasy O Smelly O Food Particles O Other_____

GRATITUDES ...TODAY I AM GRATEFUL FOR...

1._____
_____
_____
2._____
_____
_____
3._____
_____
_____

LAST NIGHT I SLEPT... _____ HOURS

○ Like a Rock   ○ Restless   ○ Difficulty Falling Asleep

○ Woke up tired   ○ Woke in the night   ○ Woke 2-3 times

...TODAY I ATE...

AM FOOD & DRINK

_____

_____

_____

_____

_____

_____

_____

_____

MID-DAY FOOD & DRINK

_____

_____

_____

_____

_____

_____

_____

...TODAY I FEEL...

MORNING MOOD

_____

_____

_____

_____

_____

AFTERNOON MOOD

_____

_____

_____

_____

_____

PM FOOD & DRINK

_____
_____
_____
_____
_____
_____
_____

EVENING MOOD

😃 🙂 😐 🙁 😢
😮 😕 😑 😣 😴

_____
_____
_____
_____
_____
_____

ELIMINATION ...EVERYBODY POOPS...

○ 1 Time   ○ 2 Times   ○ 3 Times   ○ More than 3 Times

○ Rabbit-like ○ Tootsie Roll ○ Banana-like ○ Mushy ○ Watery

○ Greasy ○ Smelly ○ Food Particles ○ Other_____

GRATITUDES ...TODAY I AM GRATEFUL FOR...

1. _____
_____
_____
2. _____
_____
_____
3. _____
_____
_____

LAST NIGHT I SLEPT...

_____ HOURS

○ Like a Rock   ○ Restless   ○ Difficulty Falling Asleep

○ Woke up tired   ○ Woke in the night ○ Woke 2-3 times

...TODAY I ATE...

AM FOOD & DRINK

_____
_____
_____
_____
_____
_____
_____
_____

MID-DAY FOOD & DRINK

_____
_____
_____
_____
_____
_____

...TODAY I FEEL...

MORNING MOOD

_____
_____
_____
_____
_____

AFTERNOON MOOD

_____
_____
_____
_____
_____

TODAY'S DATE: _____

PM FOOD & DRINK

_____
_____
_____
_____
_____
_____
_____
_____

EVENING MOOD

(☺) (☺) (☺) (☹) (☹)

(☺) (☺) (☺) (☹) (zz)

_____
_____
_____
_____
_____

ELIMINATION   ...EVERYBODY POOPS...

○ 1 Time   ○ 2 Times   ○ 3 Times   ○ More than 3 Times

○ Rabbit-like ○ Tootsie Roll ○ Banana-like ○ Mushy ○ Watery

○ Greasy ○ Smelly ○ Food Particles ○ Other_____

GRATITUDES   ...TODAY I AM GRATEFUL FOR...

1._____
_____
_____
2._____
_____
_____
3._____
_____
_____

FOOD | MOOD | GRATITUDE

LAST NIGHT I SLEPT...   _____ HOURS

○ Like a Rock   ○ Restless   ○ Difficulty Falling Asleep

○ Woke up tired   ○ Woke in the night   ○ Woke 2-3 times

...TODAY I ATE...

AM FOOD & DRINK

_____

_____

_____

_____

_____

_____

_____

MID-DAY FOOD & DRINK

_____

_____

_____

_____

_____

_____

_____

...TODAY I FEEL...

MORNING MOOD

_____

_____

_____

_____

AFTERNOON MOOD

_____

_____

_____

_____

_____

TODAY'S DATE: _____

PM FOOD & DRINK

_____
_____
_____
_____
_____
_____
_____

EVENING MOOD

_____
_____
_____
_____

ELIMINATION ...EVERYBODY POOPS...

O 1 Time   O 2 Times   O 3 Times   O More than 3 Times

O Rabbit-like O Tootsie Roll O Banana-like O Mushy O Watery

O Greasy O Smelly O Food Particles O Other_____

GRATITUDES ...TODAY I AM GRATEFUL FOR...

1. _____
_____
_____

2. _____
_____
_____

3. _____
_____
_____

FOOD | MOOD | GRATITUDE

LAST NIGHT I SLEPT... _____ HOURS

○ Like a Rock   ○ Restless   ○ Difficulty Falling Asleep

○ Woke up tired   ○ Woke in the night   ○ Woke 2-3 times

...TODAY I ATE...   ...TODAY I FEEL...

AM FOOD & DRINK

_____
_____
_____
_____
_____
_____
_____
_____
_____

MORNING MOOD

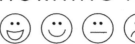

_____
_____
_____
_____
_____

MID-DAY FOOD & DRINK

_____
_____
_____
_____
_____
_____
_____
_____

AFTERNOON MOOD

_____
_____
_____
_____
_____
_____

HAPPYWELLLIFESTYLE.COM

PM FOOD & DRINK

_____
_____
_____
_____
_____
_____
_____
_____

EVENING MOOD

😀 🙂 😐 🙁 😫

😮 😕 😕 😣 😴

_____
_____
_____
_____
_____
_____

ELIMINATION   ...EVERYBODY POOPS...

○ 1 Time   ○ 2 Times   ○ 3 Times   ○ More than 3 Times

○ Rabbit-like ○ Tootsie Roll ○ Banana-like ○ Mushy ○ Watery

○ Greasy ○ Smelly ○ Food Particles ○ Other_____

GRATITUDES   ...TODAY I AM GRATEFUL FOR...

1. _____
_____
_____

2. _____
_____
_____

3. _____
_____
_____

LAST NIGHT I SLEPT... _____ HOURS

O Like a Rock   O Restless   O Difficulty Falling Asleep

O Woke up tired   O Woke in the night   O Woke 2-3 times

...TODAY I ATE...

AM FOOD & DRINK

_____
_____
_____
_____
_____
_____
_____
_____
_____

MID-DAY FOOD & DRINK

_____
_____
_____
_____
_____
_____
_____

...TODAY I FEEL...

MORNING MOOD

_____
_____
_____
_____
_____

AFTERNOON MOOD

_____
_____
_____
_____
_____

TODAY'S DATE: _____

PM FOOD & DRINK

_____
_____
_____
_____
_____
_____
_____
_____

EVENING MOOD

_____
_____
_____
_____
_____
_____

ELIMINATION   ...EVERYBODY POOPS...

O 1 Time   O 2 Times   O 3 Times   O More than 3 Times

O Rabbit-like O Tootsie Roll O Banana-like O Mushy O Watery

O Greasy O Smelly O Food Particles O Other_____

GRATITUDES   ...TODAY I AM GRATEFUL FOR...

1._____
_____
_____

2._____
_____
_____

3._____
_____
_____

FOOD | MOOD | GRATITUDE   53

LAST NIGHT I SLEPT... _____ HOURS

○ Like a Rock   ○ Restless   ○ Difficulty Falling Asleep

○ Woke up tired   ○ Woke in the night   ○ Woke 2-3 times

...TODAY I ATE...

AM FOOD & DRINK

_____
_____
_____
_____
_____
_____
_____
_____

MID-DAY FOOD & DRINK

_____
_____
_____
_____
_____
_____

...TODAY I FEEL...

MORNING MOOD

_____
_____
_____
_____
_____

AFTERNOON MOOD

_____
_____
_____
_____
_____

TODAY'S DATE: _____

PM FOOD & DRINK

_____
_____
_____
_____
_____
_____
_____
_____

EVENING MOOD

😃 🙂 😐 🙁 😫
😮 😌 😕 😣 💤

_____
_____
_____
_____
_____

ELIMINATION   ...EVERYBODY POOPS...

○ 1 Time   ○ 2 Times   ○ 3 Times   ○ More than 3 Times

○ Rabbit-like ○ Tootsie Roll ○ Banana-like ○ Mushy ○ Watery

○ Greasy ○ Smelly ○ Food Particles ○ Other_____

GRATITUDES   ...TODAY I AM GRATEFUL FOR...

1._____
_____
_____

2._____
_____
_____

3._____
_____
_____

FOOD | MOOD | GRATITUDE

LAST NIGHT I SLEPT... _____ HOURS

O Like a Rock   O Restless   O Difficulty Falling Asleep

O Woke up tired   O Woke in the night   O Woke 2-3 times

...TODAY I ATE...   ...TODAY I FEEL...

AM FOOD & DRINK

_____
_____
_____
_____
_____
_____
_____

MORNING MOOD

_____
_____
_____

MID-DAY FOOD & DRINK

_____
_____
_____
_____
_____

AFTERNOON MOOD

_____
_____
_____

TODAY'S DATE: _____

PM FOOD & DRINK

_____
_____
_____
_____
_____
_____
_____
_____
_____

EVENING MOOD

😃 🙂 😐 🙁 😢

😮 😌 😕 😣 😴

_____
_____
_____
_____
_____
_____

ELIMINATION   ...EVERYBODY POOPS...

○ 1 Time   ○ 2 Times   ○ 3 Times   ○ More than 3 Times

○ Rabbit-like ○ Tootsie Roll ○ Banana-like ○ Mushy ○ Watery

○ Greasy ○ Smelly ○ Food Particles ○ Other_____

GRATITUDES   ...TODAY I AM GRATEFUL FOR...

1._____
_____
_____

2._____
_____
_____

3._____
_____
_____

FOOD | MOOD | GRATITUDE

LAST NIGHT I SLEPT... _____ HOURS

O Like a Rock   O Restless   O Difficulty Falling Asleep

O Woke up tired   O Woke in the night   O Woke 2-3 times

...TODAY I ATE...   ...TODAY I FEEL...

AM FOOD & DRINK

_____
_____
_____
_____
_____
_____
_____
_____

MORNING MOOD

☺ ☺ ☺ ☹ ☹

☺ ☺ ☺ ☹ zz

_____
_____
_____
_____
_____

MID-DAY FOOD & DRINK

_____
_____
_____
_____
_____
_____
_____

AFTERNOON MOOD

☺ ☺ ☺ ☹ ☹

☺ ☺ ☺ ☹ zz

_____
_____
_____
_____
_____

HAPPYWELLLIFESTYLE.COM

TODAY'S DATE: _____

PM FOOD & DRINK

_____
_____
_____
_____
_____
_____
_____

EVENING MOOD

😃 🙂 😐 ☹️ 😧

😮 😌 😕 😣 😴

_____
_____
_____
_____
_____

ELIMINATION   ...EVERYBODY POOPS...

O 1 Time   O 2 Times   O 3 Times   O More than 3 Times

O Rabbit-like O Tootsie Roll O Banana-like O Mushy O Watery

O Greasy O Smelly O Food Particles O Other_____

GRATITUDES   ...TODAY I AM GRATEFUL FOR...

1._____
_____
_____

2._____
_____
_____

3._____
_____
_____

LAST NIGHT I SLEPT...   _____ HOURS

○ Like a Rock   ○ Restless   ○ Difficulty Falling Asleep

○ Woke up tired   ○ Woke in the night   ○ Woke 2-3 times

...TODAY I ATE...   ...TODAY I FEEL...

AM FOOD & DRINK   ### MORNING MOOD

_____   _____
_____   _____
_____   _____
_____   _____
_____   _____
_____   _____
_____   _____
_____   _____

MID-DAY FOOD & DRINK   ### AFTERNOON MOOD

_____   _____
_____   _____
_____   _____
_____   _____
_____   _____
_____   _____
_____   _____
_____   _____

TODAY'S DATE: _____

PM FOOD & DRINK

_____
_____
_____
_____
_____
_____
_____

EVENING MOOD

😃 🙂 😐 ☹️ 😫
😮 😕 😕 😣 😴

_____
_____
_____
_____
_____

ELIMINATION ...EVERYBODY POOPS...

O 1 Time   O 2 Times   O 3 Times   O More than 3 Times

O Rabbit-like O Tootsie Roll O Banana-like O Mushy O Watery

O Greasy O Smelly O Food Particles O Other_____

GRATITUDES ...TODAY I AM GRATEFUL FOR...

1._____
_____
_____

2._____
_____
_____

3._____
_____
_____

FOOD | MOOD | GRATITUDE

LAST NIGHT I SLEPT... _____ HOURS

O Like a Rock   O Restless   O Difficulty Falling Asleep

O Woke up tired   O Woke in the night   O Woke 2-3 times

...TODAY I ATE...

AM FOOD & DRINK

_____
_____
_____
_____
_____
_____
_____
_____

MID-DAY FOOD & DRINK

_____
_____
_____
_____
_____
_____
_____

...TODAY I FEEL...

MORNING MOOD

_____
_____
_____
_____

AFTERNOON MOOD

_____
_____
_____
_____

TODAY'S DATE: _____

PM FOOD & DRINK

_____
_____
_____
_____
_____
_____
_____
_____

EVENING MOOD

_____
_____
_____
_____
_____
_____

ELIMINATION   ...EVERYBODY POOPS...

○ 1 Time   ○ 2 Times   ○ 3 Times   ○ More than 3 Times

○ Rabbit-like ○ Tootsie Roll ○ Banana-like ○ Mushy ○ Watery

○ Greasy ○ Smelly ○ Food Particles ○ Other_____

GRATITUDES   ...TODAY I AM GRATEFUL FOR...

1._____
_____
_____

2._____
_____
_____

3._____
_____
_____

FOOD | MOOD | GRATITUDE   63

LAST NIGHT I SLEPT... _____ HOURS

○ Like a Rock   ○ Restless   ○ Difficulty Falling Asleep

○ Woke up tired   ○ Woke in the night   ○ Woke 2-3 times

...TODAY I ATE...

AM FOOD & DRINK

_____
_____
_____
_____
_____
_____
_____
_____
_____

MID-DAY FOOD & DRINK

_____
_____
_____
_____
_____
_____
_____

...TODAY I FEEL...

MORNING MOOD

_____
_____
_____
_____
_____

AFTERNOON MOOD

_____
_____
_____
_____
_____

TODAY'S DATE: _____

PM FOOD & DRINK

_____
_____
_____
_____
_____
_____
_____
_____

EVENING MOOD

😃 🙂 😐 ☹️ 😧

😮 😌 😕 😣 💤

_____
_____
_____
_____
_____

ELIMINATION   ...EVERYBODY POOPS...

O 1 Time   O 2 Times   O 3 Times   O More than 3 Times

O Rabbit-like O Tootsie Roll O Banana-like O Mushy O Watery

O Greasy O Smelly O Food Particles O Other_____

GRATITUDES   ...TODAY I AM GRATEFUL FOR...

1._____
_____
_____

2._____
_____
_____

3._____
_____
_____

FOOD | MOOD | GRATITUDE

LAST NIGHT I SLEPT... _____ HOURS

○ Like a Rock   ○ Restless   ○ Difficulty Falling Asleep

○ Woke up tired   ○ Woke in the night   ○ Woke 2-3 times

...TODAY I ATE...

...TODAY I FEEL...

AM FOOD & DRINK

MORNING MOOD

_____

_____

_____

_____

_____

_____

_____

_____

MID-DAY FOOD & DRINK

AFTERNOON MOOD

_____

_____

_____

_____

_____

_____

_____

_____

HAPPYWELLLIFESTYLE.COM

TODAY'S DATE: _____

PM FOOD & DRINK

_____
_____
_____
_____
_____
_____
_____
_____

EVENING MOOD

😃 🙂 😐 🙁 😫
😮 😕 😑 😣 😴

_____
_____
_____
_____
_____

ELIMINATION   ...EVERYBODY POOPS...

○ 1 Time   ○ 2 Times   ○ 3 Times   ○ More than 3 Times

○ Rabbit-like ○ Tootsie Roll ○ Banana-like ○ Mushy ○ Watery

○ Greasy ○ Smelly ○ Food Particles ○ Other_____

GRATITUDES   ...TODAY I AM GRATEFUL FOR...

1._____
_____
_____

2._____
_____
_____

3._____
_____
_____

FOOD | MOOD | GRATITUDE   67

LAST NIGHT I SLEPT... _____ HOURS

○ Like a Rock   ○ Restless   ○ Difficulty Falling Asleep

○ Woke up tired   ○ Woke in the night   ○ Woke 2-3 times

...TODAY I ATE...

AM FOOD & DRINK

_____
_____
_____
_____
_____
_____
_____
_____
_____

MID-DAY FOOD & DRINK

_____
_____
_____
_____
_____
_____
_____
_____

...TODAY I FEEL...

MORNING MOOD

_____
_____
_____
_____
_____
_____

AFTERNOON MOOD

_____
_____
_____
_____
_____
_____

TODAY'S DATE: _____

PM FOOD & DRINK

_____
_____
_____
_____
_____
_____
_____
_____

EVENING MOOD

☺ ☺ 😐 ☹ 😢
😮 😐 😕 😣 😴

_____
_____
_____
_____
_____

ELIMINATION   ...EVERYBODY POOPS...

○ 1 Time   ○ 2 Times   ○ 3 Times   ○ More than 3 Times

○ Rabbit-like ○ Tootsie Roll ○ Banana-like ○ Mushy ○ Watery

○ Greasy ○ Smelly ○ Food Particles ○ Other_____

GRATITUDES   ...TODAY I AM GRATEFUL FOR...

1. _____
_____
_____

2. _____
_____
_____

3. _____
_____
_____

FOOD | MOOD | GRATITUDE   69

LAST NIGHT I SLEPT... _____ HOURS

O Like a Rock   O Restless   O Difficulty Falling Asleep

O Woke up tired   O Woke in the night   O Woke 2-3 times

...TODAY I ATE...   ...TODAY I FEEL...

AM FOOD & DRINK

_____
_____
_____
_____
_____
_____
_____

MORNING MOOD

_____
_____
_____
_____

MID-DAY FOOD & DRINK

_____
_____
_____
_____
_____
_____

AFTERNOON MOOD

_____
_____
_____
_____

TODAY'S DATE: _____

PM FOOD & DRINK

_____
_____
_____
_____
_____
_____
_____

EVENING MOOD

😃 🙂 😐 🙁 😫

😲 😌 😕 😖 😴

_____
_____
_____
_____
_____
_____

ELIMINATION ...EVERYBODY POOPS...

○ 1 Time ○ 2 Times ○ 3 Times ○ More than 3 Times

○ Rabbit-like ○ Tootsie Roll ○ Banana-like ○ Mushy ○ Watery

○ Greasy ○ Smelly ○ Food Particles ○ Other_____

GRATITUDES ...TODAY I AM GRATEFUL FOR...

1._____
_____
_____

2._____
_____
_____

3._____
_____
_____

LAST NIGHT I SLEPT...   _____ HOURS

○ Like a Rock   ○ Restless   ○ Difficulty Falling Asleep

○ Woke up tired   ○ Woke in the night   ○ Woke 2-3 times

...TODAY I ATE...   ...TODAY I FEEL...

AM FOOD & DRINK

_____

_____

_____

_____

_____

_____

_____

_____

MORNING MOOD

_____

_____

_____

_____

_____

_____

MID-DAY FOOD & DRINK

_____

_____

_____

_____

_____

_____

_____

AFTERNOON MOOD

_____

_____

_____

_____

_____

_____

72   HAPPYWELLLIFESTYLE.COM

TODAY'S DATE: _____

PM FOOD & DRINK

_____
_____
_____
_____
_____
_____
_____

EVENING MOOD

😃 🙂 😐 🙁 😫

😮 😕 😕 😣 😴

_____
_____
_____
_____
_____

ELIMINATION   ...EVERYBODY POOPS...

O 1 Time   O 2 Times   O 3 Times   O More than 3 Times

O Rabbit-like O Tootsie Roll O Banana-like O Mushy O Watery

O Greasy O Smelly O Food Particles O Other_____

GRATITUDES   ...TODAY I AM GRATEFUL FOR...

1. _____
_____
_____
2. _____
_____
_____
3. _____
_____
_____

FOOD | MOOD | GRATITUDE

REVIEW YOUR MONTH: CLUES & NOTES

REVIEW YOUR MONTH: CLUES & NOTES

MONTH TWO

FUN FACT:

25 tons

...the amount of food

we ingest in our lifetime.

We are what we digest and absorb.

LAST NIGHT I SLEPT... _____ HOURS

O Like a Rock   O Restless   O Difficulty Falling Asleep

O Woke up tired   O Woke in the night   O Woke 2-3 times

...TODAY I ATE...

AM FOOD & DRINK

_____
_____
_____
_____
_____
_____
_____
_____

...TODAY I FEEL...

MORNING MOOD

_____
_____
_____
_____
_____

MID-DAY FOOD & DRINK

_____
_____
_____
_____
_____
_____
_____
_____

AFTERNOON MOOD

_____
_____
_____
_____
_____

TODAY'S DATE: _____

PM FOOD & DRINK

_____
_____
_____
_____
_____
_____
_____
_____

EVENING MOOD

😄 🙂 😐 ☹️ 😧

😮 😕 😕 😣 💤

_____
_____
_____
_____
_____

ELIMINATION ...EVERYBODY POOPS...

○ 1 Time ○ 2 Times ○ 3 Times ○ More than 3 Times

○ Rabbit-like ○ Tootsie Roll ○ Banana-like ○ Mushy ○ Watery

○ Greasy ○ Smelly ○ Food Particles ○ Other_____

GRATITUDES ...TODAY I AM GRATEFUL FOR...

1._____
_____
_____

2._____
_____
_____

3._____
_____
_____

FOOD | MOOD | GRATITUDE

LAST NIGHT I SLEPT... _____ HOURS

○ Like a Rock   ○ Restless   ○ Difficulty Falling Asleep

○ Woke up tired   ○ Woke in the night   ○ Woke 2-3 times

...TODAY I ATE...   ...TODAY I FEEL...

AM FOOD & DRINK

_____

_____

_____

_____

_____

_____

_____

_____

MORNING MOOD

_____

_____

_____

_____

_____

MID-DAY FOOD & DRINK

_____

_____

_____

_____

_____

_____

_____

_____

AFTERNOON MOOD

_____

_____

_____

_____

_____

TODAY'S DATE: _____

PM FOOD & DRINK

_____
_____
_____
_____
_____
_____
_____
_____

EVENING MOOD

😀 🙂 😐 🙁 😢
😮 😊 😕 😣 😴

_____
_____
_____
_____
_____

ELIMINATION   ...EVERYBODY POOPS...

○ 1 Time   ○ 2 Times   ○ 3 Times   ○ More than 3 Times

○ Rabbit-like ○ Tootsie Roll ○ Banana-like ○ Mushy ○ Watery

○ Greasy ○ Smelly ○ Food Particles ○ Other_____

GRATITUDES   ...TODAY I AM GRATEFUL FOR...

1. _____
_____
_____
2. _____
_____
_____
3. _____
_____
_____

LAST NIGHT I SLEPT... _____ HOURS

○ Like a Rock   ○ Restless   ○ Difficulty Falling Asleep

○ Woke up tired   ○ Woke in the night   ○ Woke 2-3 times

...TODAY I ATE...

...TODAY I FEEL...

AM FOOD & DRINK

MORNING MOOD

_____
_____
_____
_____
_____
_____
_____
_____

_____
_____
_____
_____

MID-DAY FOOD & DRINK

AFTERNOON MOOD

_____
_____
_____
_____
_____
_____
_____

_____
_____
_____
_____

PM FOOD & DRINK

_____
_____
_____
_____
_____
_____
_____
_____

EVENING MOOD

😃 🙂 😐 🙁 😫

😮 😕 😬 😣 😴

_____
_____
_____
_____
_____

ELIMINATION ...EVERYBODY POOPS...

O 1 Time   O 2 Times   O 3 Times   O More than 3 Times

O Rabbit-like O Tootsie Roll O Banana-like O Mushy O Watery

O Greasy O Smelly O Food Particles O Other_____

GRATITUDES ...TODAY I AM GRATEFUL FOR...

1._____
_____
_____

2._____
_____
_____

3._____
_____
_____

LAST NIGHT I SLEPT... _____ HOURS

○ Like a Rock   ○ Restless   ○ Difficulty Falling Asleep

○ Woke up tired   ○ Woke in the night   ○ Woke 2-3 times

...TODAY I ATE...

AM FOOD & DRINK

_____
_____
_____
_____
_____
_____
_____
_____

MID-DAY FOOD & DRINK

_____
_____
_____
_____
_____
_____
_____

...TODAY I FEEL...

MORNING MOOD

_____
_____
_____
_____
_____

AFTERNOON MOOD

_____
_____
_____
_____
_____

TODAY'S DATE: _____

PM FOOD & DRINK

_____
_____
_____
_____
_____
_____
_____
_____

EVENING MOOD

_____
_____
_____
_____
_____

ELIMINATION ...EVERYBODY POOPS...

O 1 Time O 2 Times O 3 Times O More than 3 Times

O Rabbit-like O Tootsie Roll O Banana-like O Mushy O Watery

O Greasy O Smelly O Food Particles O Other_____

GRATITUDES ...TODAY I AM GRATEFUL FOR...

1._____
_____
_____

2._____
_____
_____

3._____
_____
_____

LAST NIGHT I SLEPT... _____ HOURS

○ Like a Rock   ○ Restless   ○ Difficulty Falling Asleep

○ Woke up tired   ○ Woke in the night   ○ Woke 2-3 times

...TODAY I ATE...   ...TODAY I FEEL...

AM FOOD & DRINK

_____

_____

_____

_____

_____

_____

_____

_____

MORNING MOOD

☺ ☺ 😐 ☹ 😫

😳 😌 😕 😣 zz

_____

_____

_____

_____

_____

MID-DAY FOOD & DRINK

_____

_____

_____

_____

_____

_____

_____

_____

AFTERNOON MOOD

☺ ☺ 😐 ☹ 😫

😳 😌 😕 😣 zz

_____

_____

_____

_____

_____

PM FOOD & DRINK

_____
_____
_____
_____
_____
_____
_____
_____

EVENING MOOD

😃 🙂 😐 🙁 😢

😮 😊 😕 😣 😴

_____
_____
_____
_____
_____
_____

ELIMINATION   ...EVERYBODY POOPS...

O 1 Time   O 2 Times   O 3 Times   O More than 3 Times

O Rabbit-like O Tootsie Roll O Banana-like O Mushy O Watery

O Greasy O Smelly O Food Particles O Other_____

GRATITUDES   ...TODAY I AM GRATEFUL FOR...

1._____
_____
_____

2._____
_____
_____

3._____
_____
_____

LAST NIGHT I SLEPT... _____ HOURS

○ Like a Rock   ○ Restless   ○ Difficulty Falling Asleep

○ Woke up tired   ○ Woke in the night   ○ Woke 2-3 times

...TODAY I ATE...

AM FOOD & DRINK

_____
_____
_____
_____
_____
_____
_____
_____

MID-DAY FOOD & DRINK

_____
_____
_____
_____
_____
_____
_____

...TODAY I FEEL...

MORNING MOOD

😄 🙂 😐 ☹️ 😧

😮 😌 😕 😣 😴

_____
_____
_____
_____
_____

AFTERNOON MOOD

😄 🙂 😐 ☹️ 😧

😮 😌 😕 😣 😴

_____
_____
_____
_____

PM FOOD & DRINK

_____
_____
_____
_____
_____
_____
_____
_____

EVENING MOOD

_____
_____
_____
_____
_____

ELIMINATION   ...EVERYBODY POOPS...

○ 1 Time   ○ 2 Times   ○ 3 Times   ○ More than 3 Times

○ Rabbit-like ○ Tootsie Roll ○ Banana-like ○ Mushy ○ Watery

○ Greasy ○ Smelly ○ Food Particles ○ Other_____

GRATITUDES   ...TODAY I AM GRATEFUL FOR...

1. _____
_____
_____
2. _____
_____
_____
3. _____
_____
_____

LAST NIGHT I SLEPT... _____ HOURS

O Like a Rock   O Restless   O Difficulty Falling Asleep

O Woke up tired   O Woke in the night   O Woke 2-3 times

...TODAY I ATE...

AM FOOD & DRINK

_____
_____
_____
_____
_____
_____
_____
_____

MID-DAY FOOD & DRINK

_____
_____
_____
_____
_____
_____
_____

...TODAY I FEEL...

MORNING MOOD

_____
_____
_____
_____
_____

AFTERNOON MOOD

_____
_____
_____
_____
_____

HAPPYWELLLIFESTYLE.COM

TODAY'S DATE: _____

PM FOOD & DRINK

_____
_____
_____
_____
_____
_____
_____

EVENING MOOD

_____
_____
_____
_____
_____
_____

ELIMINATION ...EVERYBODY POOPS...

O 1 Time   O 2 Times   O 3 Times   O More than 3 Times

O Rabbit-like O Tootsie Roll O Banana-like O Mushy O Watery

O Greasy O Smelly O Food Particles O Other_____

GRATITUDES ...TODAY I AM GRATEFUL FOR...

1._____
_____
_____
2._____
_____
_____
3._____
_____
_____

FOOD | MOOD | GRATITUDE   91

LAST NIGHT I SLEPT... _____ HOURS

○ Like a Rock   ○ Restless   ○ Difficulty Falling Asleep

○ Woke up tired   ○ Woke in the night   ○ Woke 2-3 times

...TODAY I ATE...

...TODAY I FEEL...

AM FOOD & DRINK

_____
_____
_____
_____
_____
_____
_____
_____
_____

MORNING MOOD

😀 🙂 😐 🙁 😢
😲 😌 😕 😣 😴

_____
_____
_____
_____
_____

MID-DAY FOOD & DRINK

_____
_____
_____
_____
_____
_____
_____
_____
_____

AFTERNOON MOOD

😀 🙂 😐 🙁 😢
😲 😌 😕 😣 😴

_____
_____
_____
_____
_____

TODAY'S DATE: _____

PM FOOD & DRINK

_____
_____
_____
_____
_____
_____
_____
_____
_____

EVENING MOOD

_____
_____
_____
_____
_____
_____

ELIMINATION   ...EVERYBODY POOPS...

O 1 Time   O 2 Times   O 3 Times   O More than 3 Times

O Rabbit-like O Tootsie Roll O Banana-like O Mushy O Watery

O Greasy O Smelly O Food Particles O Other_____

GRATITUDES   ...TODAY I AM GRATEFUL FOR...

1. _____
_____
_____

2. _____
_____
_____

3. _____
_____
_____

LAST NIGHT I SLEPT... _____ HOURS

○ Like a Rock   ○ Restless   ○ Difficulty Falling Asleep

○ Woke up tired   ○ Woke in the night   ○ Woke 2-3 times

...TODAY I ATE...

AM FOOD & DRINK

_____
_____
_____
_____
_____
_____
_____
_____

MID-DAY FOOD & DRINK

_____
_____
_____
_____
_____
_____
_____

...TODAY I FEEL...

MORNING MOOD

_____
_____
_____
_____
_____

AFTERNOON MOOD

_____
_____
_____
_____
_____

94

TODAY'S DATE: _____

PM FOOD & DRINK

_____
_____
_____
_____
_____
_____
_____
_____

EVENING MOOD

_____
_____
_____
_____
_____

ELIMINATION   ...EVERYBODY POOPS...

O 1 Time   O 2 Times   O 3 Times   O More than 3 Times

O Rabbit-like O Tootsie Roll O Banana-like O Mushy O Watery

O Greasy O Smelly O Food Particles O Other_____

GRATITUDES   ...TODAY I AM GRATEFUL FOR...

1._____
_____
_____

2._____
_____
_____

3._____
_____
_____

LAST NIGHT I SLEPT... _____ HOURS

O Like a Rock   O Restless   O Difficulty Falling Asleep

O Woke up tired   O Woke in the night   O Woke 2-3 times

...TODAY I ATE...   ...TODAY I FEEL...

AM FOOD & DRINK

_____
_____
_____
_____
_____
_____
_____

MORNING MOOD

_____
_____
_____
_____

MID-DAY FOOD & DRINK

_____
_____
_____
_____
_____
_____
_____

AFTERNOON MOOD

_____
_____
_____
_____

TODAY'S DATE: _____

PM FOOD & DRINK

_____
_____
_____
_____
_____
_____
_____

EVENING MOOD

😃 🙂 😐 🙁 😫
😦 😕 😑 😣 😴

_____
_____
_____
_____
_____

ELIMINATION   ...EVERYBODY POOPS...

○ 1 Time   ○ 2 Times   ○ 3 Times   ○ More than 3 Times

○ Rabbit-like ○ Tootsie Roll ○ Banana-like ○ Mushy ○ Watery

○ Greasy ○ Smelly ○ Food Particles ○ Other_____

GRATITUDES   ...TODAY I AM GRATEFUL FOR...

1._____

_____

_____

2._____

_____

_____

3._____

_____

_____

FOOD | MOOD | GRATITUDE   97

LAST NIGHT I SLEPT... _____ HOURS

○ Like a Rock   ○ Restless   ○ Difficulty Falling Asleep

○ Woke up tired   ○ Woke in the night   ○ Woke 2-3 times

...TODAY I ATE...

AM FOOD & DRINK

_____
_____
_____
_____
_____
_____
_____

MID-DAY FOOD & DRINK

_____
_____
_____
_____
_____
_____
_____

...TODAY I FEEL...

MORNING MOOD

_____
_____
_____
_____

AFTERNOON MOOD

_____
_____
_____
_____

TODAY'S DATE: _____

PM FOOD & DRINK

_____
_____
_____
_____
_____
_____
_____

EVENING MOOD

_____
_____
_____
_____
_____

ELIMINATION ...EVERYBODY POOPS...

O 1 Time   O 2 Times   O 3 Times   O More than 3 Times

O Rabbit-like O Tootsie Roll O Banana-like O Mushy O Watery

O Greasy O Smelly O Food Particles O Other_____

GRATITUDES ...TODAY I AM GRATEFUL FOR...

1._____
_____
_____
2._____
_____
_____
3._____
_____
_____

FOOD | MOOD | GRATITUDE

LAST NIGHT I SLEPT...   _____ HOURS

○ Like a Rock   ○ Restless   ○ Difficulty Falling Asleep

○ Woke up tired   ○ Woke in the night   ○ Woke 2-3 times

...TODAY I ATE...

AM FOOD & DRINK

_____
_____
_____
_____
_____
_____
_____
_____

MID-DAY FOOD & DRINK

_____
_____
_____
_____
_____
_____
_____

...TODAY I FEEL...

MORNING MOOD

_____
_____
_____
_____

AFTERNOON MOOD

_____
_____
_____
_____

HAPPYWELLLIFESTYLE.COM

PM FOOD & DRINK

_____
_____
_____
_____
_____
_____
_____
_____

EVENING MOOD

_____
_____
_____
_____
_____
_____

ELIMINATION   ...EVERYBODY POOPS...

O 1 Time   O 2 Times   O 3 Times   O More than 3 Times

O Rabbit-like O Tootsie Roll O Banana-like O Mushy O Watery

O Greasy O Smelly O Food Particles O Other_____

GRATITUDES   ...TODAY I AM GRATEFUL FOR...

1._____
_____
_____

2._____
_____
_____

3._____
_____
_____

LAST NIGHT I SLEPT... _____ HOURS

○ Like a Rock   ○ Restless   ○ Difficulty Falling Asleep

○ Woke up tired   ○ Woke in the night   ○ Woke 2-3 times

...TODAY I ATE...

AM FOOD & DRINK

_____
_____
_____
_____
_____
_____
_____
_____

MID-DAY FOOD & DRINK

_____
_____
_____
_____
_____
_____
_____

...TODAY I FEEL...

MORNING MOOD

😀 🙂 😐 🙁 😫
😳 😌 😕 😣 💤

_____
_____
_____
_____
_____

AFTERNOON MOOD

😀 🙂 😐 🙁 😫
😳 😌 😕 😣 💤

_____
_____
_____
_____
_____

TODAY'S DATE: _____

PM FOOD & DRINK

_____
_____
_____
_____
_____
_____
_____
_____
_____

EVENING MOOD

😀 🙂 😐 🙁 😫
😲 😵 😕 😣 😴

_____
_____
_____
_____
_____

ELIMINATION ...EVERYBODY POOPS...

○ 1 Time ○ 2 Times ○ 3 Times ○ More than 3 Times

○ Rabbit-like ○ Tootsie Roll ○ Banana-like ○ Mushy ○ Watery

○ Greasy ○ Smelly ○ Food Particles ○ Other_____

GRATITUDES ...TODAY I AM GRATEFUL FOR...

1._____
_____
_____
2._____
_____
_____
3._____
_____
_____

LAST NIGHT I SLEPT... _____ HOURS

○ Like a Rock   ○ Restless   ○ Difficulty Falling Asleep

○ Woke up tired   ○ Woke in the night   ○ Woke 2-3 times

...TODAY I ATE...

AM FOOD & DRINK

_____

_____

_____

_____

_____

_____

_____

_____

MID-DAY FOOD & DRINK

_____

_____

_____

_____

_____

_____

_____

_____

...TODAY I FEEL...

MORNING MOOD

😃 🙂 😐 🙁 😢
😳 😕 😖 😣 😴

_____

_____

_____

_____

_____

AFTERNOON MOOD

😃 🙂 😐 🙁 😢
😳 😕 😖 😣 😴

_____

_____

_____

_____

_____

TODAY'S DATE: _____

PM FOOD & DRINK

_____
_____
_____
_____
_____
_____
_____
_____
_____

EVENING MOOD

😀 🙂 😐 🙁 😢

😮 😌 😕 😣 😴

_____
_____
_____
_____
_____

ELIMINATION   ...EVERYBODY POOPS...

O 1 Time   O 2 Times   O 3 Times   O More than 3 Times

O Rabbit-like O Tootsie Roll O Banana-like O Mushy O Watery

O Greasy O Smelly O Food Particles O Other_____

GRATITUDES   ...TODAY I AM GRATEFUL FOR...

1. _____
_____

2. _____
_____

3. _____
_____

LAST NIGHT I SLEPT... _____ HOURS

O Like a Rock   O Restless   O Difficulty Falling Asleep

O Woke up tired   O Woke in the night   O Woke 2-3 times

...TODAY I ATE...

AM FOOD & DRINK

_____
_____
_____
_____
_____
_____
_____
_____

MID-DAY FOOD & DRINK

_____
_____
_____
_____
_____
_____
_____

...TODAY I FEEL...

MORNING MOOD

_____
_____
_____
_____
_____
_____

AFTERNOON MOOD

_____
_____
_____
_____
_____
_____

HAPPYWELLLIFESTYLE.COM

PM FOOD & DRINK

_____
_____
_____
_____
_____
_____
_____
_____

EVENING MOOD

😄 🙂 😐 🙁 😢
😮 😕 😐 😣 😴

_____
_____
_____
_____
_____
_____

ELIMINATION ...EVERYBODY POOPS...

○ 1 Time   ○ 2 Times   ○ 3 Times   ○ More than 3 Times

○ Rabbit-like ○ Tootsie Roll ○ Banana-like ○ Mushy ○ Watery

○ Greasy ○ Smelly ○ Food Particles ○ Other_____

GRATITUDES ...TODAY I AM GRATEFUL FOR...

1._____
_____
_____

2._____
_____
_____

3._____
_____
_____

LAST NIGHT I SLEPT...   _____ HOURS

○ Like a Rock   ○ Restless   ○ Difficulty Falling Asleep

○ Woke up tired   ○ Woke in the night   ○ Woke 2-3 times

...TODAY I ATE...

AM FOOD & DRINK

_____

_____

_____

_____

_____

_____

_____

_____

MID-DAY FOOD & DRINK

_____

_____

_____

_____

_____

_____

_____

...TODAY I FEEL...

MORNING MOOD

_____

_____

_____

_____

_____

AFTERNOON MOOD

_____

_____

_____

_____

_____

HAPPYWELLLIFESTYLE.COM

PM FOOD & DRINK

_____
_____
_____
_____
_____
_____
_____
_____

EVENING MOOD

😃 🙂 😐 ☹️ 😰

😮 😌 😕 😣 😴

_____
_____
_____
_____
_____

ELIMINATION ...EVERYBODY POOPS...

○ 1 Time ○ 2 Times ○ 3 Times ○ More than 3 Times

○ Rabbit-like ○ Tootsie Roll ○ Banana-like ○ Mushy ○ Watery

○ Greasy ○ Smelly ○ Food Particles ○ Other_____

GRATITUDES ...TODAY I AM GRATEFUL FOR...

1._____
_____
_____

2._____
_____
_____

3._____
_____
_____

LAST NIGHT I SLEPT... _____ HOURS

O Like a Rock   O Restless   O Difficulty Falling Asleep

O Woke up tired   O Woke in the night   O Woke 2-3 times

...TODAY I ATE...

AM FOOD & DRINK

_____
_____
_____
_____
_____
_____
_____
_____

MID-DAY FOOD & DRINK

_____
_____
_____
_____
_____
_____
_____

...TODAY I FEEL...

MORNING MOOD

_____
_____
_____
_____
_____

AFTERNOON MOOD

_____
_____
_____
_____
_____

HAPPYWELLLIFESTYLE.COM

TODAY'S DATE: _____

PM FOOD & DRINK

_____
_____
_____
_____
_____
_____
_____
_____

EVENING MOOD

(☺) (☺) (😐) (☹) (😢)
(😮) (😕) (😕) (😣) (zz)

_____
_____
_____
_____
_____
_____

ELIMINATION ...EVERYBODY POOPS...

○ 1 Time   ○ 2 Times   ○ 3 Times   ○ More than 3 Times

○ Rabbit-like ○ Tootsie Roll ○ Banana-like ○ Mushy ○ Watery

○ Greasy ○ Smelly ○ Food Particles ○ Other_____

GRATITUDES ...TODAY I AM GRATEFUL FOR...

1._____
_____
_____

2._____
_____
_____

3._____
_____
_____

LAST NIGHT I SLEPT... _____ HOURS

O Like a Rock   O Restless   O Difficulty Falling Asleep

O Woke up tired   O Woke in the night   O Woke 2-3 times

...TODAY I ATE...

AM FOOD & DRINK

_____
_____
_____
_____
_____
_____
_____
_____
_____

MID-DAY FOOD & DRINK

_____
_____
_____
_____
_____
_____
_____
_____

...TODAY I FEEL...

MORNING MOOD

_____
_____
_____
_____
_____
_____

AFTERNOON MOOD

_____
_____
_____
_____
_____
_____

PM FOOD & DRINK

_____
_____
_____
_____
_____
_____
_____
_____

EVENING MOOD

😃 🙂 😐 🙁 😫

😮 😕 😐 😣 😴

_____
_____
_____
_____
_____

ELIMINATION ...EVERYBODY POOPS...

○ 1 Time   ○ 2 Times   ○ 3 Times   ○ More than 3 Times

○ Rabbit-like ○ Tootsie Roll ○ Banana-like ○ Mushy ○ Watery

○ Greasy ○ Smelly ○ Food Particles ○ Other_____

GRATITUDES   ...TODAY I AM GRATEFUL FOR...

1._____
_____
_____

2._____
_____
_____

3._____
_____
_____

LAST NIGHT I SLEPT... _____ HOURS

○ Like a Rock ○ Restless ○ Difficulty Falling Asleep

○ Woke up tired ○ Woke in the night ○ Woke 2-3 times

...TODAY I ATE...   ...TODAY I FEEL...

AM FOOD & DRINK

_____
_____
_____
_____
_____
_____
_____

MORNING MOOD

_____
_____
_____
_____
_____

MID-DAY FOOD & DRINK

_____
_____
_____
_____
_____
_____

AFTERNOON MOOD

_____
_____
_____
_____

TODAY'S DATE: _____

PM FOOD & DRINK

_____
_____
_____
_____
_____
_____
_____
_____

EVENING MOOD

😀 🙂 😐 ☹️ 😩
😮 😌 😕 😣 💤

_____
_____
_____
_____
_____

ELIMINATION ...EVERYBODY POOPS...

○ 1 Time ○ 2 Times ○ 3 Times ○ More than 3 Times

○ Rabbit-like ○ Tootsie Roll ○ Banana-like ○ Mushy ○ Watery

○ Greasy ○ Smelly ○ Food Particles ○ Other_____

GRATITUDES ...TODAY I AM GRATEFUL FOR...

1._____
_____
_____

2._____
_____
_____

3._____
_____
_____

FOOD | MOOD | GRATITUDE   115

LAST NIGHT I SLEPT... _____ HOURS

○ Like a Rock   ○ Restless   ○ Difficulty Falling Asleep

○ Woke up tired   ○ Woke in the night   ○ Woke 2-3 times

...TODAY I ATE...   ...TODAY I FEEL...

AM FOOD & DRINK

_____
_____
_____
_____
_____
_____
_____
_____

MORNING MOOD

_____
_____
_____
_____

MID-DAY FOOD & DRINK

_____
_____
_____
_____
_____
_____

AFTERNOON MOOD

_____
_____
_____
_____

HAPPYWELLLIFESTYLE.COM

TODAY'S DATE: _____

PM FOOD & DRINK

_____
_____
_____
_____
_____
_____
_____
_____

EVENING MOOD

😄 🙂 😐 🙁 😢
😮 😬 😕 😣 😴

_____
_____
_____
_____
_____

ELIMINATION ...EVERYBODY POOPS...

○ 1 Time   ○ 2 Times   ○ 3 Times   ○ More than 3 Times

○ Rabbit-like ○ Tootsie Roll ○ Banana-like ○ Mushy ○ Watery

○ Greasy ○ Smelly ○ Food Particles ○ Other_____

GRATITUDES ...TODAY I AM GRATEFUL FOR...

1. _____
_____
_____

2. _____
_____
_____

3. _____
_____
_____

FOOD | MOOD | GRATITUDE

LAST NIGHT I SLEPT... _____ HOURS

○ Like a Rock   ○ Restless   ○ Difficulty Falling Asleep

○ Woke up tired   ○ Woke in the night   ○ Woke 2-3 times

...TODAY I ATE...

AM FOOD & DRINK

_____
_____
_____
_____
_____
_____
_____
_____
_____

MID-DAY FOOD & DRINK

_____
_____
_____
_____
_____
_____
_____
_____

...TODAY I FEEL...

MORNING MOOD

_____
_____
_____
_____
_____

AFTERNOON MOOD

_____
_____
_____
_____
_____

PM FOOD & DRINK

_____
_____
_____
_____
_____
_____
_____
_____

EVENING MOOD

_____
_____
_____
_____
_____
_____

ELIMINATION   ...EVERYBODY POOPS...

O 1 Time   O 2 Times   O 3 Times   O More than 3 Times

O Rabbit-like O Tootsie Roll O Banana-like O Mushy O Watery

O Greasy O Smelly O Food Particles O Other_____

GRATITUDES   ...TODAY I AM GRATEFUL FOR...

1._____

_____

_____

2._____

_____

_____

3._____

_____

_____

LAST NIGHT I SLEPT... _____ HOURS

○ Like a Rock   ○ Restless   ○ Difficulty Falling Asleep

○ Woke up tired   ○ Woke in the night   ○ Woke 2-3 times

...TODAY I ATE...

AM FOOD & DRINK

_____

_____

_____

_____

_____

_____

_____

_____

MID-DAY FOOD & DRINK

_____

_____

_____

_____

_____

_____

_____

_____

...TODAY I FEEL...

MORNING MOOD

_____

_____

_____

_____

_____

AFTERNOON MOOD

_____

_____

_____

_____

_____

TODAY'S DATE: _____

PM FOOD & DRINK

_____
_____
_____
_____
_____
_____
_____
_____

EVENING MOOD

😃 🙂 😐 🙁 😣

😮 😕 😟 😖 😴

_____
_____
_____
_____
_____

ELIMINATION ...EVERYBODY POOPS...

○ 1 Time   ○ 2 Times   ○ 3 Times   ○ More than 3 Times

○ Rabbit-like ○ Tootsie Roll ○ Banana-like ○ Mushy ○ Watery

○ Greasy ○ Smelly ○ Food Particles ○ Other_____

GRATITUDES ...TODAY I AM GRATEFUL FOR...

1._____
_____
_____
2._____
_____
_____
3._____
_____
_____

LAST NIGHT I SLEPT...

_____ HOURS

○ Like a Rock   ○ Restless   ○ Difficulty Falling Asleep

○ Woke up tired   ○ Woke in the night   ○ Woke 2-3 times

...TODAY I ATE...

AM FOOD & DRINK

_____

_____

_____

_____

_____

_____

_____

MID-DAY FOOD & DRINK

_____

_____

_____

_____

_____

_____

_____

...TODAY I FEEL...

MORNING MOOD

_____

_____

_____

_____

AFTERNOON MOOD

_____

_____

_____

_____

TODAY'S DATE: _____

PM FOOD & DRINK

_____
_____
_____
_____
_____
_____
_____
_____

EVENING MOOD

😀 🙂 😐 🙁 😫

😦 😶 😕 😣 😴

_____
_____
_____
_____
_____
_____

ELIMINATION ...EVERYBODY POOPS...

○ 1 Time   ○ 2 Times   ○ 3 Times   ○ More than 3 Times

○ Rabbit-like ○ Tootsie Roll ○ Banana-like ○ Mushy ○ Watery

○ Greasy ○ Smelly ○ Food Particles ○ Other_____

GRATITUDES ...TODAY I AM GRATEFUL FOR...

1._____
_____
_____
2._____
_____
_____
3._____
_____
_____

LAST NIGHT I SLEPT...   _____ HOURS

○ Like a Rock   ○ Restless   ○ Difficulty Falling Asleep

○ Woke up tired   ○ Woke in the night   ○ Woke 2-3 times

...TODAY I ATE...

AM FOOD & DRINK

_____
_____
_____
_____
_____
_____
_____
_____
_____

MID-DAY FOOD & DRINK

_____
_____
_____
_____
_____
_____
_____

...TODAY I FEEL...

MORNING MOOD

_____
_____
_____
_____
_____

AFTERNOON MOOD

_____
_____
_____
_____

124   HAPPYWELLLIFESTYLE.COM

TODAY'S DATE: _____

PM FOOD & DRINK

_____
_____
_____
_____
_____
_____
_____
_____

EVENING MOOD

😃 🙂 😐 🙁 😫
😮 😕 😐 😣 💤

_____
_____
_____
_____
_____
_____

ELIMINATION   ...EVERYBODY POOPS...

○ 1 Time   ○ 2 Times   ○ 3 Times   ○ More than 3 Times

○ Rabbit-like ○ Tootsie Roll ○ Banana-like ○ Mushy ○ Watery

○ Greasy ○ Smelly ○ Food Particles ○ Other_____

GRATITUDES   ...TODAY I AM GRATEFUL FOR...

1._____
_____
_____

2._____
_____
_____

3._____
_____
_____

FOOD | MOOD | GRATITUDE

LAST NIGHT I SLEPT... _____ HOURS

O Like a Rock   O Restless   O Difficulty Falling Asleep

O Woke up tired   O Woke in the night   O Woke 2-3 times

...TODAY I ATE...   ...TODAY I FEEL...

AM FOOD & DRINK

_____
_____
_____
_____
_____
_____
_____
_____

MORNING MOOD

_____
_____
_____
_____
_____
_____

MID-DAY FOOD & DRINK

_____
_____
_____
_____
_____
_____
_____
_____

AFTERNOON MOOD

_____
_____
_____
_____
_____
_____

HAPPYWELLLIFESTYLE.COM

TODAY'S DATE: _____

PM FOOD & DRINK

_____
_____
_____
_____
_____
_____
_____
_____

EVENING MOOD

😃 🙂 😐 🙁 😣

😮 😖 😕 😤 😴

_____
_____
_____
_____
_____

ELIMINATION ...EVERYBODY POOPS...

○ 1 Time   ○ 2 Times   ○ 3 Times   ○ More than 3 Times

○ Rabbit-like ○ Tootsie Roll ○ Banana-like ○ Mushy ○ Watery

○ Greasy ○ Smelly ○ Food Particles ○ Other_____

GRATITUDES ...TODAY I AM GRATEFUL FOR...

1. _____
_____
_____

2. _____
_____
_____

3. _____
_____
_____

FOOD | MOOD | GRATITUDE

LAST NIGHT I SLEPT... _____ HOURS

○ Like a Rock   ○ Restless   ○ Difficulty Falling Asleep

○ Woke up tired   ○ Woke in the night   ○ Woke 2-3 times

...TODAY I ATE...

AM FOOD & DRINK

_____

_____

_____

_____

_____

_____

_____

MID-DAY FOOD & DRINK

_____

_____

_____

_____

_____

_____

_____

...TODAY I FEEL...

MORNING MOOD

😀 🙂 😐 🙁 😢
😳 😕 😟 😖 💤

_____

_____

_____

_____

_____

AFTERNOON MOOD

😀 🙂 😐 🙁 😢
😳 😕 😟 😖 💤

_____

_____

_____

_____

_____

HAPPYWELLLIFESTYLE.COM

TODAY'S DATE: _____

PM FOOD & DRINK

_____
_____
_____
_____
_____
_____
_____

EVENING MOOD

😃 🙂 😐 ☹️ 😢
😮 😌 😕 😣 💤

_____
_____
_____
_____
_____

ELIMINATION   ...EVERYBODY POOPS...

○ 1 Time   ○ 2 Times   ○ 3 Times   ○ More than 3 Times

○ Rabbit-like ○ Tootsie Roll ○ Banana-like ○ Mushy ○ Watery

○ Greasy ○ Smelly ○ Food Particles ○ Other_____

GRATITUDES   ...TODAY I AM GRATEFUL FOR...

1. _____
_____
_____
2. _____
_____
_____
3. _____
_____
_____

FOOD | MOOD | GRATITUDE   129

LAST NIGHT I SLEPT...   _____ HOURS

○ Like a Rock   ○ Restless   ○ Difficulty Falling Asleep

○ Woke up tired   ○ Woke in the night ○ Woke 2-3 times

...TODAY I ATE...

AM FOOD & DRINK

_____

_____

_____

_____

_____

_____

_____

_____

MID-DAY FOOD & DRINK

_____

_____

_____

_____

_____

_____

...TODAY I FEEL...

MORNING MOOD

_____

_____

_____

_____

_____

AFTERNOON MOOD

_____

_____

_____

_____

_____

TODAY'S DATE: _____

PM FOOD & DRINK

_____
_____
_____
_____
_____
_____
_____

EVENING MOOD

(:D) (:)) (:|) (:( ) (;( )

(:o) (~) (:/) (><) (zz)

_____
_____
_____
_____
_____

ELIMINATION   ...EVERYBODY POOPS...

O 1 Time   O 2 Times   O 3 Times   O More than 3 Times

O Rabbit-like O Tootsie Roll O Banana-like O Mushy O Watery

O Greasy O Smelly O Food Particles O Other_____

GRATITUDES   ...TODAY I AM GRATEFUL FOR...

1._____
_____
_____

2._____
_____
_____

3._____
_____
_____

FOOD | MOOD | GRATITUDE

LAST NIGHT I SLEPT... _____ HOURS

○ Like a Rock   ○ Restless   ○ Difficulty Falling Asleep

○ Woke up tired   ○ Woke in the night   ○ Woke 2-3 times

...TODAY I ATE...

AM FOOD & DRINK

_____
_____
_____
_____
_____
_____
_____
_____

MID-DAY FOOD & DRINK

_____
_____
_____
_____
_____
_____
_____

...TODAY I FEEL...

MORNING MOOD

_____
_____
_____
_____
_____

AFTERNOON MOOD

_____
_____
_____
_____
_____

HAPPYWELLLIFESTYLE.COM

TODAY'S DATE: _____

PM FOOD & DRINK

_____
_____
_____
_____
_____
_____
_____
_____

EVENING MOOD

_____
_____
_____
_____
_____
_____

ELIMINATION   ...EVERYBODY POOPS...

O 1 Time   O 2 Times   O 3 Times   O More than 3 Times

O Rabbit-like O Tootsie Roll O Banana-like O Mushy O Watery

O Greasy O Smelly O Food Particles O Other_____

GRATITUDES   ...TODAY I AM GRATEFUL FOR...

1. _____
_____
_____

2. _____
_____
_____

3. _____
_____
_____

LAST NIGHT I SLEPT...   _____ HOURS

○ Like a Rock   ○ Restless   ○ Difficulty Falling Asleep

○ Woke up tired   ○ Woke in the night   ○ Woke 2-3 times

...TODAY I ATE...   ...TODAY I FEEL...

AM FOOD & DRINK

_____
_____
_____
_____
_____
_____
_____
_____

MORNING MOOD

_____
_____
_____
_____

MID-DAY FOOD & DRINK

_____
_____
_____
_____
_____
_____
_____
_____

AFTERNOON MOOD

_____
_____
_____
_____

TODAY'S DATE: _____

PM FOOD & DRINK

_____
_____
_____
_____
_____
_____
_____
_____

EVENING MOOD

😀 🙂 😐 🙁 😫

😮 😕 😕 😣 😴

_____
_____
_____
_____
_____

ELIMINATION   ...EVERYBODY POOPS...

○ 1 Time   ○ 2 Times   ○ 3 Times   ○ More than 3 Times

○ Rabbit-like ○ Tootsie Roll ○ Banana-like ○ Mushy ○ Watery

○ Greasy ○ Smelly ○ Food Particles ○ Other_____

GRATITUDES   ...TODAY I AM GRATEFUL FOR...

1._____
_____
_____
2._____
_____
_____
3._____
_____
_____

FOOD | MOOD | GRATITUDE

LAST NIGHT I SLEPT... _____ HOURS

○ Like a Rock   ○ Restless   ○ Difficulty Falling Asleep

○ Woke up tired   ○ Woke in the night   ○ Woke 2-3 times

...TODAY I ATE...   ...TODAY I FEEL...

AM FOOD & DRINK

_____
_____
_____
_____
_____
_____

MORNING MOOD

_____
_____
_____
_____

MID-DAY FOOD & DRINK

_____
_____
_____
_____
_____
_____

AFTERNOON MOOD

_____
_____
_____
_____

PM FOOD & DRINK

_____
_____
_____
_____
_____
_____
_____
_____

EVENING MOOD

😃 🙂 😐 🙁 😫

😮 😕 😕 😣 😴

_____
_____
_____
_____
_____
_____

ELIMINATION   ...EVERYBODY POOPS...

○ 1 Time   ○ 2 Times   ○ 3 Times   ○ More than 3 Times

○ Rabbit-like ○ Tootsie Roll ○ Banana-like ○ Mushy ○ Watery

○ Greasy ○ Smelly ○ Food Particles ○ Other_____

GRATITUDES   ...TODAY I AM GRATEFUL FOR...

1._____
_____
_____
2._____
_____
_____
3._____
_____
_____

LAST NIGHT I SLEPT...   _____ HOURS

○ Like a Rock   ○ Restless   ○ Difficulty Falling Asleep

○ Woke up tired   ○ Woke in the night   ○ Woke 2-3 times

...TODAY I ATE...

AM FOOD & DRINK

_____
_____
_____
_____
_____
_____
_____
_____

MID-DAY FOOD & DRINK

_____
_____
_____
_____
_____
_____
_____
_____

...TODAY I FEEL...

MORNING MOOD

_____
_____
_____
_____
_____

AFTERNOON MOOD

_____
_____
_____
_____
_____

TODAY'S DATE: _____

PM FOOD & DRINK

_____
_____
_____
_____
_____
_____
_____
_____
_____

EVENING MOOD

😃 🙂 😐 🙁 😫
😮 😌 😕 😣 😴

_____
_____
_____
_____
_____
_____

ELIMINATION   ...EVERYBODY POOPS...

○ 1 Time   ○ 2 Times   ○ 3 Times   ○ More than 3 Times

○ Rabbit-like ○ Tootsie Roll ○ Banana-like ○ Mushy ○ Watery

○ Greasy ○ Smelly ○ Food Particles ○ Other_____

GRATITUDES   ...TODAY I AM GRATEFUL FOR...

1. _____
_____
_____

2. _____
_____
_____

3. _____
_____
_____

REVIEW YOUR MONTH: CLUES & NOTES

REVIEW YOUR MONTH: CLUES & NOTES

_____
_____
_____
_____
_____
_____
_____
_____
_____
_____
_____
_____
_____
_____
_____
_____
_____
_____
_____
_____
_____
_____
_____
_____
_____
_____
_____
_____

MONTH
THREE

FUN FACT:

¹/₃ cup

...the amount of added sugar most Americans
consume on a daily basis. Excess sugar
of any kind is stored as belly fat.

LAST NIGHT I SLEPT... _____ HOURS

O Like a Rock   O Restless   O Difficulty Falling Asleep

O Woke up tired   O Woke in the night   O Woke 2-3 times

...TODAY I ATE...   ...TODAY I FEEL...

AM FOOD & DRINK

_____

_____

_____

_____

_____

_____

_____

_____

MORNING MOOD

MID-DAY FOOD & DRINK

_____

_____

_____

_____

_____

_____

AFTERNOON MOOD

TODAY'S DATE: _____

PM FOOD & DRINK

_____
_____
_____
_____
_____
_____
_____
_____

EVENING MOOD

☺ ☺ ☺ ☹ ☹
☺ ☺ ☺ ☹ zz

_____
_____
_____
_____
_____

ELIMINATION   ...EVERYBODY POOPS...

○ 1 Time   ○ 2 Times   ○ 3 Times   ○ More than 3 Times

○ Rabbit-like ○ Tootsie Roll ○ Banana-like ○ Mushy ○ Watery

○ Greasy ○ Smelly ○ Food Particles ○ Other_____

GRATITUDES   ...TODAY I AM GRATEFUL FOR...

1._____
_____
_____

2._____
_____
_____

3._____
_____
_____

FOOD | MOOD | GRATITUDE

LAST NIGHT I SLEPT... _____ HOURS

○ Like a Rock   ○ Restless   ○ Difficulty Falling Asleep

○ Woke up tired   ○ Woke in the night   ○ Woke 2-3 times

...TODAY I ATE...

AM FOOD & DRINK

_____
_____
_____
_____
_____
_____
_____
_____

MID-DAY FOOD & DRINK

_____
_____
_____
_____
_____
_____
_____

...TODAY I FEEL...

MORNING MOOD

_____
_____
_____
_____
_____
_____

AFTERNOON MOOD

_____
_____
_____
_____
_____
_____

     HAPPYWELLLIFESTYLE.COM

TODAY'S DATE: _____

PM FOOD & DRINK

_____
_____
_____
_____
_____
_____
_____
_____
_____

EVENING MOOD

😄 🙂 😐 🙁 😢

😮 😌 😕 😣 😴

_____
_____
_____
_____
_____
_____

ELIMINATION   ...EVERYBODY POOPS...

○ 1 Time   ○ 2 Times   ○ 3 Times   ○ More than 3 Times

○ Rabbit-like ○ Tootsie Roll ○ Banana-like ○ Mushy ○ Watery

○ Greasy ○ Smelly ○ Food Particles ○ Other_____

GRATITUDES   ...TODAY I AM GRATEFUL FOR...

1._____
_____
_____
2._____
_____
_____
3._____
_____
_____

LAST NIGHT I SLEPT... _____ HOURS

○ Like a Rock   ○ Restless   ○ Difficulty Falling Asleep

○ Woke up tired   ○ Woke in the night   ○ Woke 2-3 times

...TODAY I ATE...

AM FOOD & DRINK

_____
_____
_____
_____
_____
_____
_____
_____

MID-DAY FOOD & DRINK

_____
_____
_____
_____
_____
_____
_____

...TODAY I FEEL...

MORNING MOOD

_____
_____
_____
_____
_____

AFTERNOON MOOD

_____
_____
_____
_____
_____

HAPPYWELLLIFESTYLE.COM

PM FOOD & DRINK

_____
_____
_____
_____
_____
_____
_____
_____

EVENING MOOD

_____
_____
_____
_____
_____
_____

ELIMINATION   ...EVERYBODY POOPS...

O 1 Time   O 2 Times   O 3 Times   O More than 3 Times

O Rabbit-like O Tootsie Roll O Banana-like O Mushy O Watery

O Greasy O Smelly O Food Particles O Other_____

GRATITUDES   ...TODAY I AM GRATEFUL FOR...

1._____
_____
_____
2._____
_____
_____
3._____
_____
_____

LAST NIGHT I SLEPT... _____ HOURS

○ Like a Rock   ○ Restless   ○ Difficulty Falling Asleep

○ Woke up tired   ○ Woke in the night   ○ Woke 2-3 times

...TODAY I ATE...

...TODAY I FEEL...

AM FOOD & DRINK

MORNING MOOD

_____
_____
_____
_____
_____
_____
_____
_____
_____

_____
_____
_____
_____
_____
_____

MID-DAY FOOD & DRINK

AFTERNOON MOOD

_____
_____
_____
_____
_____
_____
_____
_____
_____

_____
_____
_____
_____
_____
_____

HAPPYWELLLIFESTYLE.COM

TODAY'S DATE: _____

PM FOOD & DRINK

_____
_____
_____
_____
_____
_____
_____
_____

EVENING MOOD

😃 🙂 😐 🙁 😰

😮 😕 😕 😣 😴

_____
_____
_____
_____
_____

ELIMINATION ...EVERYBODY POOPS...

○ 1 Time   ○ 2 Times   ○ 3 Times   ○ More than 3 Times

○ Rabbit-like ○ Tootsie Roll ○ Banana-like ○ Mushy ○ Watery

○ Greasy ○ Smelly ○ Food Particles ○ Other_____

GRATITUDES ...TODAY I AM GRATEFUL FOR...

1. _____
_____
_____
2. _____
_____
_____
3. _____
_____
_____

LAST NIGHT I SLEPT... _____ HOURS

○ Like a Rock   ○ Restless   ○ Difficulty Falling Asleep

○ Woke up tired   ○ Woke in the night   ○ Woke 2-3 times

...TODAY I ATE...   ...TODAY I FEEL...

AM FOOD & DRINK

_____

_____

_____

_____

_____

_____

_____

_____

MORNING MOOD

_____

_____

_____

_____

_____

MID-DAY FOOD & DRINK

_____

_____

_____

_____

_____

_____

_____

_____

AFTERNOON MOOD

_____

_____

_____

_____

_____

HAPPYWELLLIFESTYLE.COM

TODAY'S DATE: _____

PM FOOD & DRINK

_____
_____
_____
_____
_____
_____
_____
_____

EVENING MOOD

😃 🙂 😐 🙁 😰

😮 😌 😕 😣 💤

_____
_____
_____
_____
_____
_____

ELIMINATION   ...EVERYBODY POOPS...

O 1 Time   O 2 Times   O 3 Times   O More than 3 Times

O Rabbit-like O Tootsie Roll O Banana-like O Mushy O Watery

O Greasy O Smelly O Food Particles O Other_____

GRATITUDES   ...TODAY I AM GRATEFUL FOR...

1._____
_____
_____
2._____
_____
_____
3._____
_____
_____

LAST NIGHT I SLEPT...   _____ HOURS

○ Like a Rock   ○ Restless   ○ Difficulty Falling Asleep

○ Woke up tired   ○ Woke in the night   ○ Woke 2-3 times

...TODAY I ATE...

AM FOOD & DRINK

_____

_____

_____

_____

_____

_____

_____

_____

MID-DAY FOOD & DRINK

_____

_____

_____

_____

_____

_____

...TODAY I FEEL...

MORNING MOOD

_____

_____

_____

_____

_____

AFTERNOON MOOD

_____

_____

_____

_____

_____

HAPPYWELLLIFESTYLE.COM

TODAY'S DATE: _____

PM FOOD & DRINK

_____
_____
_____
_____
_____
_____
_____

EVENING MOOD

_____
_____
_____
_____
_____
_____

ELIMINATION ...EVERYBODY POOPS...

O 1 Time   O 2 Times   O 3 Times   O More than 3 Times

O Rabbit-like O Tootsie Roll O Banana-like O Mushy O Watery

O Greasy O Smelly O Food Particles O Other_____

GRATITUDES ...TODAY I AM GRATEFUL FOR...

1._____
_____
_____
2._____
_____
_____
3._____
_____
_____

FOOD | MOOD | GRATITUDE   155

LAST NIGHT I SLEPT... _____ HOURS

O Like a Rock   O Restless   O Difficulty Falling Asleep

O Woke up tired   O Woke in the night   O Woke 2-3 times

...TODAY I ATE...   ...TODAY I FEEL...

AM FOOD & DRINK

_____
_____
_____
_____
_____
_____

MORNING MOOD

MID-DAY FOOD & DRINK

_____
_____
_____
_____
_____

AFTERNOON MOOD

PM FOOD & DRINK

_____
_____
_____
_____
_____
_____
_____
_____
_____

EVENING MOOD

😃 🙂 😐 🙁 �«

😮 😕 😬 😣 😴

_____
_____
_____
_____
_____
_____

ELIMINATION ...EVERYBODY POOPS...

O 1 Time   O 2 Times   O 3 Times   O More than 3 Times

O Rabbit-like O Tootsie Roll O Banana-like O Mushy O Watery

O Greasy O Smelly O Food Particles O Other_____

GRATITUDES ...TODAY I AM GRATEFUL FOR...

1._____

_____

_____

2._____

_____

_____

3._____

_____

_____

LAST NIGHT I SLEPT... _____ HOURS

○ Like a Rock   ○ Restless   ○ Difficulty Falling Asleep

○ Woke up tired   ○ Woke in the night   ○ Woke 2-3 times

...TODAY I ATE...

AM FOOD & DRINK

_____

_____

_____

_____

_____

_____

_____

MID-DAY FOOD & DRINK

_____

_____

_____

_____

_____

_____

_____

...TODAY I FEEL...

MORNING MOOD

_____

_____

_____

_____

_____

AFTERNOON MOOD

_____

_____

_____

_____

_____

TODAY'S DATE: _____

PM FOOD & DRINK

_____
_____
_____
_____
_____
_____
_____
_____

EVENING MOOD

😃 🙂 😐 🙁 😖

😮 😕 😬 😣 😴

_____
_____
_____
_____
_____
_____

ELIMINATION   ...EVERYBODY POOPS...

○ 1 Time   ○ 2 Times   ○ 3 Times   ○ More than 3 Times

○ Rabbit-like ○ Tootsie Roll ○ Banana-like ○ Mushy ○ Watery

○ Greasy ○ Smelly ○ Food Particles ○ Other_____

GRATITUDES   ...TODAY I AM GRATEFUL FOR...

1._____
_____
_____
2._____
_____
_____
3._____
_____
_____

LAST NIGHT I SLEPT... _____ HOURS

○ Like a Rock   ○ Restless   ○ Difficulty Falling Asleep

○ Woke up tired   ○ Woke in the night   ○ Woke 2-3 times

...TODAY I ATE...

...TODAY I FEEL...

AM FOOD & DRINK

MORNING MOOD

_____

_____

_____

_____

_____

_____

_____

_____

MID-DAY FOOD & DRINK

AFTERNOON MOOD

_____

_____

_____

_____

_____

_____

_____

HAPPYWELLLIFESTYLE.COM

TODAY'S DATE: _____

PM FOOD & DRINK

_____
_____
_____
_____
_____
_____
_____
_____

EVENING MOOD

_____
_____
_____
_____
_____
_____

ELIMINATION   ...EVERYBODY POOPS...

○ 1 Time   ○ 2 Times   ○ 3 Times   ○ More than 3 Times

○ Rabbit-like ○ Tootsie Roll ○ Banana-like ○ Mushy ○ Watery

○ Greasy ○ Smelly ○ Food Particles ○ Other_____

GRATITUDES   ...TODAY I AM GRATEFUL FOR...

1._____
_____
_____

2._____
_____
_____

3._____
_____
_____

FOOD | MOOD | GRATITUDE

LAST NIGHT I SLEPT...   _____ HOURS

O Like a Rock   O Restless   O Difficulty Falling Asleep

O Woke up tired   O Woke in the night   O Woke 2-3 times

...TODAY I ATE...   ...TODAY I FEEL...

AM FOOD & DRINK

MORNING MOOD

_____

_____

_____

_____

_____

_____

_____

_____

MID-DAY FOOD & DRINK

AFTERNOON MOOD

_____

_____

_____

_____

_____

_____

_____

_____

PM FOOD & DRINK

_____
_____
_____
_____
_____
_____
_____
_____

EVENING MOOD

😃 🙂 😐 🙁 😢

😮 😌 😕 😣 😴

_____
_____
_____
_____
_____
_____

ELIMINATION ...EVERYBODY POOPS...

○ 1 Time   ○ 2 Times   ○ 3 Times   ○ More than 3 Times

○ Rabbit-like ○ Tootsie Roll ○ Banana-like ○ Mushy ○ Watery

○ Greasy ○ Smelly ○ Food Particles ○ Other_____

GRATITUDES ...TODAY I AM GRATEFUL FOR...

1._____
_____
_____
2._____
_____
_____
3._____
_____
_____

LAST NIGHT I SLEPT... _____ HOURS

O Like a Rock   O Restless   O Difficulty Falling Asleep

O Woke up tired   O Woke in the night   O Woke 2-3 times

...TODAY I ATE...   ...TODAY I FEEL...

AM FOOD & DRINK

_____
_____
_____
_____
_____
_____
_____
_____

MORNING MOOD

_____
_____
_____
_____
_____

MID-DAY FOOD & DRINK

_____
_____
_____
_____
_____
_____
_____
_____

AFTERNOON MOOD

_____
_____
_____
_____
_____

HAPPYWELLLIFESTYLE.COM

PM FOOD & DRINK

_____
_____
_____
_____
_____
_____
_____

EVENING MOOD

_____
_____
_____
_____
_____
_____

ELIMINATION   ...EVERYBODY POOPS...

○ 1 Time   ○ 2 Times   ○ 3 Times   ○ More than 3 Times

○ Rabbit-like ○ Tootsie Roll ○ Banana-like ○ Mushy ○ Watery

○ Greasy ○ Smelly ○ Food Particles ○ Other_____

GRATITUDES   ...TODAY I AM GRATEFUL FOR...

1. _____
_____
_____

2. _____
_____
_____

3. _____
_____
_____

LAST NIGHT I SLEPT... _____ HOURS

O Like a Rock   O Restless   O Difficulty Falling Asleep

O Woke up tired   O Woke in the night   O Woke 2-3 times

...TODAY I ATE...   ...TODAY I FEEL...

AM FOOD & DRINK

_____
_____
_____
_____
_____
_____
_____
_____

MORNING MOOD

_____
_____
_____
_____
_____

MID-DAY FOOD & DRINK

_____
_____
_____
_____
_____
_____
_____

AFTERNOON MOOD

_____
_____
_____
_____
_____

HAPPYWELLLIFESTYLE.COM

TODAY'S DATE: _____

PM FOOD & DRINK

_____
_____
_____
_____
_____
_____
_____

EVENING MOOD

😃 🙂 😐 🙁 😢
😮 😕 😐 😣 😴

_____
_____
_____
_____

ELIMINATION   ...EVERYBODY POOPS...

○ 1 Time   ○ 2 Times   ○ 3 Times   ○ More than 3 Times

○ Rabbit-like ○ Tootsie Roll ○ Banana-like ○ Mushy ○ Watery

○ Greasy ○ Smelly ○ Food Particles ○ Other_____

GRATITUDES   ...TODAY I AM GRATEFUL FOR...

1. _____
_____
_____

2. _____
_____
_____

3. _____
_____
_____

FOOD | MOOD | GRATITUDE

LAST NIGHT I SLEPT... _____ HOURS

○ Like a Rock   ○ Restless   ○ Difficulty Falling Asleep
○ Woke up tired   ○ Woke in the night   ○ Woke 2-3 times

...TODAY I ATE...

AM FOOD & DRINK

_____
_____
_____
_____
_____
_____
_____
_____

MID-DAY FOOD & DRINK

_____
_____
_____
_____
_____
_____
_____

...TODAY I FEEL...

MORNING MOOD

_____
_____
_____
_____
_____

AFTERNOON MOOD

_____
_____
_____
_____
_____

TODAY'S DATE: _____

PM FOOD & DRINK

_____
_____
_____
_____
_____
_____
_____
_____

EVENING MOOD

😃 🙂 😐 🙁 😫
😮 😕 😟 😣 😴

_____
_____
_____
_____
_____
_____

ELIMINATION ...EVERYBODY POOPS...

○ 1 Time ○ 2 Times ○ 3 Times ○ More than 3 Times

○ Rabbit-like ○ Tootsie Roll ○ Banana-like ○ Mushy ○ Watery

○ Greasy ○ Smelly ○ Food Particles ○ Other_____

GRATITUDES ...TODAY I AM GRATEFUL FOR...

1._____
_____
_____

2._____
_____
_____

3._____
_____
_____

LAST NIGHT I SLEPT...   _____ HOURS

○ Like a Rock   ○ Restless   ○ Difficulty Falling Asleep

○ Woke up tired   ○ Woke in the night   ○ Woke 2-3 times

...TODAY I ATE...   ...TODAY I FEEL...

AM FOOD & DRINK   ### MORNING MOOD

_____

_____

_____

_____

_____

_____

_____

_____

MID-DAY FOOD & DRINK   ### AFTERNOON MOOD

_____

_____

_____

_____

_____

_____

_____

TODAY'S DATE: _____

PM FOOD & DRINK

_____
_____
_____
_____
_____
_____
_____
_____

EVENING MOOD

😀 🙂 😐 🙁 😰

😮 😌 😕 😖 😴

_____
_____
_____
_____
_____
_____

ELIMINATION ...EVERYBODY POOPS...

O 1 Time   O 2 Times   O 3 Times   O More than 3 Times

O Rabbit-like O Tootsie Roll O Banana-like O Mushy O Watery

O Greasy O Smelly O Food Particles O Other_____

GRATITUDES ...TODAY I AM GRATEFUL FOR...

1._____
_____
_____
2._____
_____
_____
3._____
_____
_____

LAST NIGHT I SLEPT... _____ HOURS

○ Like a Rock   ○ Restless   ○ Difficulty Falling Asleep
○ Woke up tired   ○ Woke in the night   ○ Woke 2-3 times

...TODAY I ATE...   ...TODAY I FEEL...

AM FOOD & DRINK

_____
_____
_____
_____
_____
_____
_____
_____
_____

MORNING MOOD

_____
_____
_____
_____
_____
_____

MID-DAY FOOD & DRINK

_____
_____
_____
_____
_____
_____
_____
_____
_____

AFTERNOON MOOD

_____
_____
_____
_____
_____
_____

HAPPYWELLLIFESTYLE.COM

TODAY'S DATE: _____

PM FOOD & DRINK

_____
_____
_____
_____
_____
_____
_____

EVENING MOOD

😃 🙂 😐 🙁 😫

😮 😕 😕 😣 😴

_____
_____
_____
_____
_____

ELIMINATION ...EVERYBODY POOPS...

○ 1 Time ○ 2 Times ○ 3 Times ○ More than 3 Times

○ Rabbit-like ○ Tootsie Roll ○ Banana-like ○ Mushy ○ Watery

○ Greasy ○ Smelly ○ Food Particles ○ Other_____

GRATITUDES ...TODAY I AM GRATEFUL FOR...

1. _____
_____
_____

2. _____
_____
_____

3. _____
_____
_____

FOOD | MOOD | GRATITUDE

LAST NIGHT I SLEPT... _____ HOURS

○ Like a Rock   ○ Restless   ○ Difficulty Falling Asleep

○ Woke up tired   ○ Woke in the night   ○ Woke 2-3 times

...TODAY I ATE...   ...TODAY I FEEL...

AM FOOD & DRINK

_____
_____
_____
_____
_____
_____
_____
_____
_____

MORNING MOOD

_____
_____
_____
_____
_____

MID-DAY FOOD & DRINK

_____
_____
_____
_____
_____
_____
_____
_____

AFTERNOON MOOD

_____
_____
_____
_____

HAPPYWELLLIFESTYLE.COM

PM FOOD & DRINK

_____
_____
_____
_____
_____
_____
_____
_____

EVENING MOOD

😃 🙂 😐 ☹️ 😧

😮 😌 😕 😣 💤

_____
_____
_____
_____
_____

ELIMINATION   ...EVERYBODY POOPS...

○ 1 Time   ○ 2 Times   ○ 3 Times   ○ More than 3 Times

○ Rabbit-like ○ Tootsie Roll ○ Banana-like ○ Mushy ○ Watery

○ Greasy ○ Smelly ○ Food Particles ○ Other_____

GRATITUDES   ...TODAY I AM GRATEFUL FOR...

1._____
_____
_____
2._____
_____
_____
3._____
_____
_____

LAST NIGHT I SLEPT...

_____ HOURS

○ Like a Rock   ○ Restless   ○ Difficulty Falling Asleep

○ Woke up tired   ○ Woke in the night   ○ Woke 2-3 times

...TODAY I ATE...

AM FOOD & DRINK

_____
_____
_____
_____
_____
_____
_____
_____

MID-DAY FOOD & DRINK

_____
_____
_____
_____
_____
_____
_____
_____

...TODAY I FEEL...

MORNING MOOD

_____
_____
_____
_____
_____

AFTERNOON MOOD

_____
_____
_____
_____
_____

HAPPYWELLLIFESTYLE.COM

TODAY'S DATE: _____

PM FOOD & DRINK

_____
_____
_____
_____
_____
_____
_____
_____

EVENING MOOD

😃 🙂 😐 🙁 😢

😮 😌 😕 😣 💤

_____
_____
_____
_____
_____

ELIMINATION   ...EVERYBODY POOPS...

O 1 Time   O 2 Times   O 3 Times   O More than 3 Times

O Rabbit-like O Tootsie Roll O Banana-like O Mushy O Watery

O Greasy O Smelly O Food Particles O Other_____

GRATITUDES   ...TODAY I AM GRATEFUL FOR...

1. _____
_____
_____

2. _____
_____
_____

3. _____
_____
_____

FOOD | MOOD | GRATITUDE

LAST NIGHT I SLEPT... _____ HOURS

○ Like a Rock ○ Restless ○ Difficulty Falling Asleep

○ Woke up tired ○ Woke in the night ○ Woke 2-3 times

...TODAY I ATE...

AM FOOD & DRINK

_____

_____

_____

_____

_____

_____

_____

_____

...TODAY I FEEL...

MORNING MOOD

_____

_____

_____

_____

_____

MID-DAY FOOD & DRINK

_____

_____

_____

_____

_____

_____

_____

_____

AFTERNOON MOOD

_____

_____

_____

_____

_____

HAPPYWELLLIFESTYLE.COM

TODAY'S DATE: _____

PM FOOD & DRINK

_____
_____
_____
_____
_____
_____
_____

EVENING MOOD

😃 🙂 😐 🙁 😢

😮 😌 😕 😣 😴

_____
_____
_____
_____
_____

ELIMINATION   ...EVERYBODY POOPS...

○ 1 Time   ○ 2 Times   ○ 3 Times   ○ More than 3 Times

○ Rabbit-like ○ Tootsie Roll ○ Banana-like ○ Mushy ○ Watery

○ Greasy ○ Smelly ○ Food Particles ○ Other_____

GRATITUDES   ...TODAY I AM GRATEFUL FOR...

1._____
_____
_____

2._____
_____
_____

3._____
_____
_____

FOOD | MOOD | GRATITUDE

LAST NIGHT I SLEPT...   _____ HOURS

O Like a Rock   O Restless   O Difficulty Falling Asleep

O Woke up tired   O Woke in the night   O Woke 2-3 times

...TODAY I ATE...   ...TODAY I FEEL...

AM FOOD & DRINK   ## MORNING MOOD

_____

_____

_____

_____

_____

_____

_____

_____

MID-DAY FOOD & DRINK   ## AFTERNOON MOOD

_____

_____

_____

_____

_____

_____

_____

TODAY'S DATE: _____

PM FOOD & DRINK

_____
_____
_____
_____
_____
_____
_____
_____

EVENING MOOD

😃 🙂 😐 🙁 😧

😮 😕 😟 😣 😴

_____
_____
_____
_____
_____

ELIMINATION ...EVERYBODY POOPS...

○ 1 Time ○ 2 Times ○ 3 Times ○ More than 3 Times

○ Rabbit-like ○ Tootsie Roll ○ Banana-like ○ Mushy ○ Watery

○ Greasy ○ Smelly ○ Food Particles ○ Other_____

GRATITUDES ...TODAY I AM GRATEFUL FOR...

1. _____
_____
_____

2. _____
_____
_____

3. _____
_____
_____

FOOD | MOOD | GRATITUDE

LAST NIGHT I SLEPT... _____ HOURS

○ Like a Rock   ○ Restless   ○ Difficulty Falling Asleep

○ Woke up tired   ○ Woke in the night   ○ Woke 2-3 times

...TODAY I ATE...

AM FOOD & DRINK

_____

_____

_____

_____

_____

_____

_____

_____

MID-DAY FOOD & DRINK

_____

_____

_____

_____

_____

_____

_____

...TODAY I FEEL...

MORNING MOOD

_____

_____

_____

_____

_____

AFTERNOON MOOD

_____

_____

_____

_____

_____

HAPPYWELLLIFESTYLE.COM

TODAY'S DATE: _____

PM FOOD & DRINK

_____
_____
_____
_____
_____
_____
_____
_____
_____

EVENING MOOD

😀 🙂 😐 🙁 😫
😮 😕 😌 😣 💤

_____
_____
_____
_____
_____
_____

ELIMINATION   ...EVERYBODY POOPS...

O 1 Time   O 2 Times   O 3 Times   O More than 3 Times

O Rabbit-like O Tootsie Roll O Banana-like O Mushy O Watery

O Greasy O Smelly O Food Particles O Other_____

GRATITUDES   ...TODAY I AM GRATEFUL FOR...

1._____
_____
_____

2._____
_____
_____

3._____
_____
_____

LAST NIGHT I SLEPT...   _____ HOURS

○ Like a Rock   ○ Restless   ○ Difficulty Falling Asleep

○ Woke up tired   ○ Woke in the night   ○ Woke 2-3 times

...TODAY I ATE...   ...TODAY I FEEL...

AM FOOD & DRINK   ## MORNING MOOD

_____   😀 🙂 😐 🙁 😫

_____   😮 😌 😕 😣 😴

_____

_____   _____

_____   _____

_____   _____

_____   _____

_____   _____

MID-DAY FOOD & DRINK   ## AFTERNOON MOOD

_____   😀 🙂 😐 🙁 😫

_____   😮 😌 😕 😣 😴

_____

_____   _____

_____   _____

_____   _____

_____   _____

_____   _____

184

PM FOOD & DRINK

_____
_____
_____
_____
_____
_____
_____
_____

EVENING MOOD

😃 😊 😐 🙁 😢

😮 😋 😕 😣 😴

_____
_____
_____
_____
_____

ELIMINATION ...EVERYBODY POOPS...

○ 1 Time   ○ 2 Times   ○ 3 Times   ○ More than 3 Times

○ Rabbit-like ○ Tootsie Roll ○ Banana-like ○ Mushy ○ Watery

○ Greasy ○ Smelly ○ Food Particles ○ Other_____

GRATITUDES ...TODAY I AM GRATEFUL FOR...

1._____
_____
_____
2._____
_____
_____
3._____
_____
_____

FOOD | MOOD | GRATITUDE

LAST NIGHT I SLEPT...

_____ HOURS

○ Like a Rock   ○ Restless   ○ Difficulty Falling Asleep

○ Woke up tired   ○ Woke in the night   ○ Woke 2-3 times

...TODAY I ATE...

AM FOOD & DRINK

_____
_____
_____
_____
_____
_____
_____
_____
_____

MID-DAY FOOD & DRINK

_____
_____
_____
_____
_____
_____
_____
_____

...TODAY I FEEL...

MORNING MOOD

_____
_____
_____
_____
_____
_____

AFTERNOON MOOD

_____
_____
_____
_____
_____

TODAY'S DATE: _____

PM FOOD & DRINK

_____
_____
_____
_____
_____
_____
_____
_____

EVENING MOOD

_____
_____
_____
_____
_____
_____

ELIMINATION ...EVERYBODY POOPS...

○ 1 Time   ○ 2 Times   ○ 3 Times   ○ More than 3 Times

○ Rabbit-like ○ Tootsie Roll ○ Banana-like ○ Mushy ○ Watery

○ Greasy ○ Smelly ○ Food Particles ○ Other_____

GRATITUDES ...TODAY I AM GRATEFUL FOR...

1._____
_____
_____
2._____
_____
_____
3._____
_____
_____

FOOD | MOOD | GRATITUDE

LAST NIGHT I SLEPT... _____ HOURS

○ Like a Rock   ○ Restless   ○ Difficulty Falling Asleep

○ Woke up tired   ○ Woke in the night   ○ Woke 2-3 times

...TODAY I ATE...

AM FOOD & DRINK

_____
_____
_____
_____
_____
_____
_____
_____
_____

MID-DAY FOOD & DRINK

_____
_____
_____
_____
_____
_____
_____
_____

...TODAY I FEEL...

MORNING MOOD

_____
_____
_____
_____
_____
_____
_____

AFTERNOON MOOD

_____
_____
_____
_____
_____
_____

TODAY'S DATE: _____

PM FOOD & DRINK

_____
_____
_____
_____
_____
_____
_____
_____

EVENING MOOD

😃 🙂 😐 🙁 😨

😯 😊 😕 😣 💤

_____
_____
_____
_____
_____

ELIMINATION   ...EVERYBODY POOPS...

O 1 Time   O 2 Times   O 3 Times   O More than 3 Times

O Rabbit-like O Tootsie Roll O Banana-like O Mushy O Watery

O Greasy O Smelly O Food Particles O Other_____

GRATITUDES   ...TODAY I AM GRATEFUL FOR...

1._____
_____
_____
2._____
_____
_____
3._____
_____
_____

LAST NIGHT I SLEPT... _____ HOURS

○ Like a Rock   ○ Restless   ○ Difficulty Falling Asleep

○ Woke up tired   ○ Woke in the night   ○ Woke 2-3 times

...TODAY I ATE...   ...TODAY I FEEL...

AM FOOD & DRINK

_____
_____
_____
_____
_____
_____
_____
_____

MORNING MOOD

😃 🙂 😐 🙁 😫
😮 😕 😐 😣 💤

_____
_____
_____
_____
_____

MID-DAY FOOD & DRINK

_____
_____
_____
_____
_____
_____
_____
_____

AFTERNOON MOOD

😃 🙂 😐 🙁 😫
😮 😕 😐 😣 💤

_____
_____
_____
_____
_____

TODAY'S DATE: _____

PM FOOD & DRINK

_____
_____
_____
_____
_____
_____
_____
_____

EVENING MOOD

😀 🙂 😐 🙁 😢

😮 😌 😕 😣 😴

_____
_____
_____
_____
_____

ELIMINATION ...EVERYBODY POOPS...

○ 1 Time   ○ 2 Times   ○ 3 Times   ○ More than 3 Times

○ Rabbit-like ○ Tootsie Roll ○ Banana-like ○ Mushy ○ Watery

○ Greasy ○ Smelly ○ Food Particles ○ Other_____

GRATITUDES ...TODAY I AM GRATEFUL FOR...

1. _____
_____
_____

2. _____
_____
_____

3. _____
_____
_____

FOOD | MOOD | GRATITUDE   191

LAST NIGHT I SLEPT... _____ HOURS

O Like a Rock   O Restless   O Difficulty Falling Asleep

O Woke up tired   O Woke in the night   O Woke 2-3 times

...TODAY I ATE...

AM FOOD & DRINK

_____
_____
_____
_____
_____
_____
_____
_____

...TODAY I FEEL...

MORNING MOOD

_____
_____
_____
_____
_____

MID-DAY FOOD & DRINK

_____
_____
_____
_____
_____
_____
_____
_____

AFTERNOON MOOD

_____
_____
_____
_____
_____

HAPPYWELLLIFESTYLE.COM

TODAY'S DATE: _____

PM FOOD & DRINK

_____
_____
_____
_____
_____
_____
_____
_____
_____

EVENING MOOD

😀 🙂 😐 🙁 😫

😯 😵 😕 😠 😴

_____
_____
_____
_____
_____

ELIMINATION ...EVERYBODY POOPS...

○ 1 Time   ○ 2 Times   ○ 3 Times   ○ More than 3 Times

○ Rabbit-like ○ Tootsie Roll ○ Banana-like ○ Mushy ○ Watery

○ Greasy ○ Smelly ○ Food Particles ○ Other_____

GRATITUDES ...TODAY I AM GRATEFUL FOR...

1._____
_____
_____

2._____
_____
_____

3._____
_____
_____

FOOD | MOOD | GRATITUDE   193

LAST NIGHT I SLEPT...   _____ HOURS

○ Like a Rock   ○ Restless   ○ Difficulty Falling Asleep

○ Woke up tired   ○ Woke in the night   ○ Woke 2-3 times

...TODAY I ATE...   ...TODAY I FEEL...

AM FOOD & DRINK

_____
_____
_____
_____
_____
_____
_____

MORNING MOOD

😀 🙂 😐 🙁 😢
😳 😕 😕 😣 💤

_____
_____
_____
_____
_____

MID-DAY FOOD & DRINK

_____
_____
_____
_____
_____
_____
_____

AFTERNOON MOOD

😀 🙂 😐 🙁 😢
😳 😕 😕 😣 💤

_____
_____
_____
_____
_____

HAPPYWELLLIFESTYLE.COM

TODAY'S DATE: _____

PM FOOD & DRINK

_____
_____
_____
_____
_____
_____
_____
_____

EVENING MOOD

_____
_____
_____
_____
_____
_____

ELIMINATION   ...EVERYBODY POOPS...

○ 1 Time   ○ 2 Times   ○ 3 Times   ○ More than 3 Times

○ Rabbit-like ○ Tootsie Roll ○ Banana-like ○ Mushy ○ Watery

○ Greasy ○ Smelly ○ Food Particles ○ Other_____

GRATITUDES   ...TODAY I AM GRATEFUL FOR...

1. _____
_____
_____

2. _____
_____
_____

3. _____
_____
_____

LAST NIGHT I SLEPT... _____ HOURS

○ Like a Rock   ○ Restless   ○ Difficulty Falling Asleep

○ Woke up tired   ○ Woke in the night   ○ Woke 2-3 times

...TODAY I ATE...   ...TODAY I FEEL...

AM FOOD & DRINK

_____
_____
_____
_____
_____
_____
_____

MORNING MOOD

_____
_____
_____
_____

MID-DAY FOOD & DRINK

_____
_____
_____
_____
_____
_____

AFTERNOON MOOD

_____
_____
_____
_____

TODAY'S DATE: _____

PM FOOD & DRINK

_____
_____
_____
_____
_____
_____
_____
_____

EVENING MOOD

😀 🙂 😐 🙁 😧

😮 😕 😬 😣 😴

_____
_____
_____
_____
_____

ELIMINATION   ...EVERYBODY POOPS...

○ 1 Time   ○ 2 Times   ○ 3 Times   ○ More than 3 Times

○ Rabbit-like ○ Tootsie Roll ○ Banana-like ○ Mushy ○ Watery

○ Greasy ○ Smelly ○ Food Particles ○ Other_____

GRATITUDES   ...TODAY I AM GRATEFUL FOR...

1. _____
_____
_____
2. _____
_____
_____
3. _____
_____
_____

LAST NIGHT I SLEPT... _____ HOURS

○ Like a Rock   ○ Restless   ○ Difficulty Falling Asleep

○ Woke up tired   ○ Woke in the night   ○ Woke 2-3 times

...TODAY I ATE...   ...TODAY I FEEL...

AM FOOD & DRINK

_____
_____
_____
_____
_____
_____
_____
_____

MORNING MOOD

☺ ☺ ☺ ☹ ☹
☺ ☺ ☺ ☹ zz

_____
_____
_____
_____
_____

MID-DAY FOOD & DRINK

_____
_____
_____
_____
_____
_____
_____

AFTERNOON MOOD

☺ ☺ ☺ ☹ ☹
☺ ☺ ☺ ☹ zz

_____
_____
_____
_____
_____

HAPPYWELLLIFESTYLE.COM

PM FOOD & DRINK

_____
_____
_____
_____
_____
_____
_____
_____

EVENING MOOD

😀 🙂 😐 🙁 😫

😮 😕 😦 😣 😴

_____
_____
_____
_____
_____
_____

ELIMINATION   ...EVERYBODY POOPS...

○ 1 Time   ○ 2 Times   ○ 3 Times   ○ More than 3 Times

○ Rabbit-like ○ Tootsie Roll ○ Banana-like ○ Mushy ○ Watery

○ Greasy ○ Smelly ○ Food Particles ○ Other_____

GRATITUDES   ...TODAY I AM GRATEFUL FOR...

1._____
_____
_____
2._____
_____
_____
3._____
_____
_____

LAST NIGHT I SLEPT...   _____ HOURS

○ Like a Rock   ○ Restless   ○ Difficulty Falling Asleep

○ Woke up tired   ○ Woke in the night   ○ Woke 2-3 times

...TODAY I ATE...

...TODAY I FEEL...

AM FOOD & DRINK

MORNING MOOD

_____

_____

_____

_____

_____

_____

_____

_____

MID-DAY FOOD & DRINK

AFTERNOON MOOD

_____

_____

_____

_____

_____

_____

_____

_____

HAPPYWELLLIFESTYLE.COM

TODAY'S DATE: _____

PM FOOD & DRINK

_____
_____
_____

_____
_____
_____
_____
_____
_____

EVENING MOOD

😃 🙂 😐 🙁 😢

😮 😕 😒 😣 😴

_____
_____
_____
_____
_____
_____

ELIMINATION   ...EVERYBODY POOPS...

O 1 Time   O 2 Times   O 3 Times   O More than 3 Times

O Rabbit-like O Tootsie Roll O Banana-like O Mushy O Watery

O Greasy O Smelly O Food Particles O Other_____

GRATITUDES   ...TODAY I AM GRATEFUL FOR...

1. _____
_____
_____

2. _____
_____
_____

3. _____
_____
_____

LAST NIGHT I SLEPT... _____ HOURS

○ Like a Rock   ○ Restless   ○ Difficulty Falling Asleep

○ Woke up tired   ○ Woke in the night   ○ Woke 2-3 times

...TODAY I ATE...   ...TODAY I FEEL...

AM FOOD & DRINK

_____
_____
_____
_____
_____
_____
_____

MORNING MOOD

_____
_____
_____
_____
_____

MID-DAY FOOD & DRINK

_____
_____
_____
_____
_____
_____
_____

AFTERNOON MOOD

_____
_____
_____
_____
_____
_____

HAPPYWELLLIFESTYLE.COM

TODAY'S DATE: _____

PM FOOD & DRINK

_____
_____
_____
_____
_____
_____
_____
_____

EVENING MOOD

_____
_____
_____
_____
_____

ELIMINATION   ...EVERYBODY POOPS...

○ 1 Time   ○ 2 Times   ○ 3 Times   ○ More than 3 Times

○ Rabbit-like ○ Tootsie Roll ○ Banana-like ○ Mushy ○ Watery

○ Greasy ○ Smelly ○ Food Particles ○ Other_____

GRATITUDES   ...TODAY I AM GRATEFUL FOR...

1._____
_____

2._____
_____

3._____
_____

LAST NIGHT I SLEPT...   _____ HOURS

O Like a Rock   O Restless   O Difficulty Falling Asleep

O Woke up tired   O Woke in the night   O Woke 2-3 times

...TODAY I ATE...   ...TODAY I FEEL...

AM FOOD & DRINK

_____
_____
_____
_____
_____
_____
_____
_____
_____

MORNING MOOD

_____
_____
_____
_____
_____
_____
_____
_____

MID-DAY FOOD & DRINK

_____
_____
_____
_____
_____
_____
_____
_____
_____

AFTERNOON MOOD

_____
_____
_____
_____
_____
_____
_____
_____

HAPPYWELLLIFESTYLE.COM

TODAY'S DATE: _____

PM FOOD & DRINK

_____
_____
_____
_____
_____
_____
_____

EVENING MOOD

😃 🙂 😐 🙁 😫
😲 😌 😕 😖 😴

_____
_____
_____
_____
_____

ELIMINATION ...EVERYBODY POOPS...

○ 1 Time   ○ 2 Times   ○ 3 Times   ○ More than 3 Times

○ Rabbit-like ○ Tootsie Roll ○ Banana-like ○ Mushy ○ Watery

○ Greasy ○ Smelly ○ Food Particles ○ Other_____

GRATITUDES ...TODAY I AM GRATEFUL FOR...

1. _____
_____
_____

2. _____
_____
_____

3. _____
_____
_____

REVIEW YOUR MONTH: CLUES & NOTES

REVIEW YOUR MONTH: CLUES & NOTES

_____
_____
_____
_____
_____
_____
_____
_____
_____
_____
_____
_____
_____
_____
_____
_____
_____
_____
_____
_____
_____
_____
_____
_____
_____
_____
_____
_____
_____

CONGRATULATIONS!

Wahoo!! You've completed ninety days of your *Food, Mood, & Gratitude Journal*!

What were your ah-ha moments? Did you get some good clues to help you create your optimal wellness plan, take charge of your health, and feel great?

Nice work! You're well on your way to living a healthier, happier, more vibrant life.

HOW CAN A HEALTH COACH HELP YOU?

Are you feeling low energy, tired, depressed, confused, or anxious? Maybe you can't fall asleep or stay asleep? Are you experiencing weight gain, bloating, gas, diarrhea, constipation, or other digestion issues? Are you bothered by chronic aches and pains?

Have you been to the doctor only to be told it's all in your head? Are you too young to feel this old? With so many medical specialists these days and *a pill for every ill*, who is looking at your WHOLE health picture? I've been there… and that's why I became a certified holistic health coach, to help others thrive in wellness.

My *Kickstart Your Health* wellness program will guide you in making dietary and lifestyle choices, hold you accountable to reaching your happiness and wellness goals, and provide lots of fun motivation along the way.

Please visit HappyWellLifestyle.com/food-mood-gratitude to learn more. Plus receive a discount when you sign up for my *Kickstart Your Health* wellness program. I look forward to working with you!

Heidi Hackler

Heidi Hackler, CHHC,
Happy Well Lifestyle

HappyWellLifesytle.com/food-mood-gratitude
instagram.com/happywelllife
facebook.com/happywelllifestyle

THANKS!

Many thanks again for your purchase. If you enjoyed this journal, please consider leaving a review on the retailer's site where you purchased the journal.

Reviews are important because they help other people make decisions about whether a book or journal is going to be right for them.

You have our thanks in advance!

The Ingenium Journals team

Ingenium Journals
Ingenium Books Publishing Inc.
Toronto, ON
Canada M6P 1Z2

ingeniumbooks.com